DATE DUE

Stress and Health Among the Elderly

May L. Wykle, PhD, RN, FAAN, is the Florence Cellar Professor of Gerontological Nursing, Frances Payne Bolton School of Nursing, Case Western Reserve University (CWRU), and chairperson in psychiatric/mental health nursing at University Hospitals of Cleveland. She is also the director of the University Center on Aging and Health, CWRU. A recipient of a National Institute of Mental Health (NIMH) Geriatric Mental Health Academic Award and director of a five-year Robert Wood Johnson Teaching Nursing Home Project, Dr. Wykle's work has been concentrated on enhancing mental health services in long-term care settings. She currently serves on the National Institute on Aging research review committee and was the 1989 recipient of the John S. Diekhoff Award for excellence in teaching at CWRU. Dr. Wykle has written numerous articles, contributing chapters, and books. Three of her most recent books are *Decision Making in Long-Term Care*, coauthored with Ruth Dunkle; *Memory, Aging, and Dementia*, written with Grover Gilmore and Peter Whitehouse; and *Practicing Rehabilitation with Geriatric Clients*, with J. Dermot Frengley and Patrick Murray as coauthors.

Eva Kahana, PhD, is the Pierce T. and Elizabeth D. Robson Professor of the Humanities, chair of the Department of Sociology, and director, Elderly Care Research Center at Case Western Reserve University. She currently serves as director of predoctoral and postdoctoral training programs in health research and aging. Dr. Kahana received her BA in political science from Stern College for Women, her MA in clinical psychology from the City College, and her PhD in human development from the University of Chicago. She also completed a postdoctoral fellowship with the Midwest Council on Social Research in Aging and was awarded a Career Scientist Development Award by NIMH. Dr. Kahana has served as chair of the Behavioral and Social Sciences section of the Gerontological Society of America (GSA) (1984–85). She is a recipient of the GSA Distinguished Mentorship Award (1987) and was elected as a life member of the Wayne State University Academy of Scholars. Dr. Kahana was named Armington Professor at CWRU for the 1989–90 academic year, and received a doctor of humane letters from Yeshiva University in 1991. A recipient of a MERIT Award from the National Institute of Aging for the study of Adaptation to Frailty Among Dispersed Elders (1989–94), Dr. Kahana has published extensively in the areas of stress, coping and health of the aged, late-life migration, and environmental influences on older persons.

Jerome Kowal, MD, received his undergraduate degree from Tufts University and his medical degree from Johns Hopkins University School of Medicine. He was on the faculty of Medicine at Mt. Sinai School of Medicine from 1965 to 1970. In 1970, Dr. Kowal joined the faculty at CWRU; he has served as professor of medicine there since 1974. He was chief of the Medical Service at the Cleveland Veterans Administration Medical Center (1974–77) and the chief of staff and associate dean for Veterans Affairs at CWRU (1977–84). More recently he has directed the Geriatric Center for Clinical Assessment, Research and Education (a joint program of the CWRU School of Medicine, University Hospitals of Cleveland, and the Cleveland Veterans Administration Medical Center). He directs the Western Reserve Geriatric Education Center, which is a consortium of three Colleges of Medicine and professional schools in Northern Ohio, and also a National Institutes of Health Research Training Fellowship Program in Aging.

STRESS AND HEALTH AMONG THE ELDERLY

May L. Wykle, PhD, RN, FAAN
Eva Kahana, PhD
Jerome Kowal, MD

Editors

SPRINGER PUBLISHING COMPANY
New York

Springer Publishing Company, Inc.
536 Broadway
New York, NY 10012-3955

92 93 94 95 96 / 5 4 3 2 1

Library of Congress Cataloging-in-Publication Data

Stress and health among the elderly / May L. Wykle, Eva Kahana, and
   Jerome Kowal, editors.
        p.   cm.
     Includes bibliographical references and index.
     ISBN 0-8261-7320-9
     1. Stress in old age.   2. Aged—Health and hygiene.
   3. Geriatrics—Psychosomatic aspects.   I. Wykle, May L.
   II. Kahana, Eva.   III. Kowal, Jerome.
     [DNLM: 1. Adaptation, Psychological—in old age.   2. Stress,
   Psychological—in old age.   WM 172 S91316]
   RC952.5.S77   1992
   618.97′698—dc20
   DNLM/DLC
   for Library of Congress   91-4873
                                                                  CIP

Printed in the United States of America

Contents

Contributors

Carolyn M. Aldwin, PhD, Assistant Professor, Human Development and Family Studies, Department of Applied Behavioral Sciences, University of California, Davis, CA

Toni C. Antonucci, PhD, Professor of Psychology and Research Scientist, Survey Research Center, Institute for Social Research, University of Michigan

Beverly A. Baldwin, PhD, RN, Associate Professor and Coordinator, Graduate Program in Gerontological Nursing, School of Nursing, University of Maryland

Pamela Brown, MSW, Director of Resident and Family Services, Iowa Jewish Senior Life Center, Demoine, Iowa

David A. Chiriboga, AB, PhD, Professor and Chair, Department of Graduate Studies, School of Allied Health Sciences, University of Texas Medical Branch

Margaret Gatz, PhD, Professor, Department of Psychology, University of Southern California

Richard W. Hubbard, PhD, Assistant Professor, Department of Medicine, Case Western Reserve University

James S. Jackson, PhD, Professor of Psychology and Research Scientist, Research Center for Group Dynamics, Institute for Social Research, University of Michigan

Boaz Kahana, PhD, Professor, Department of Psychology; Director, Center on Applied Gerontological Research, Cleveland State University

Stanislav V. Kasl, PhD, Professor of Epidemiology, Department of Epidemiology and Public Health, Yale University School of Medicine

John S. Kennedy, MD, FRCP(C), Assistant Professor of Psychiatry, Department of Psychiatry, Division of Geriatrics, School of Medicine, Case Western Reserve University

Morton A. Lieberman, PhD, Professor and Director, Aging and Mental Health Program, Department of Psychiatry, University of California at San Francisco

Joseph T. Mullan, PhD, Assistant Adjunct Professor, Department of Psychiatry, University of California at San Francisco

Leonard I. Pearlin, PhD, Professor, Department of Psychiatry, Program in Human Development and Aging, University of California at San Francisco

Thomas H. Walz, PhD, MSW, Professor, School of Social Work, University of Iowa

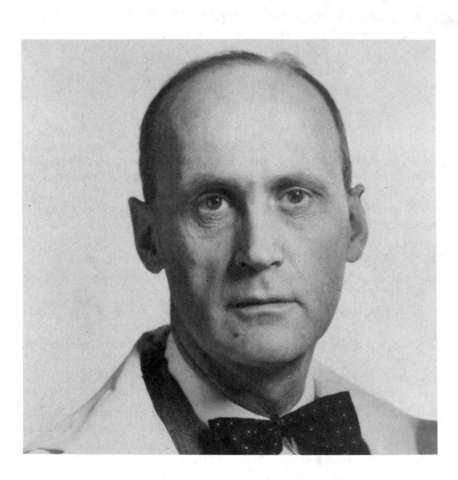

In Memoriam
Austin B. Chinn, MD (1908–1989)

Geriatric medicine and gerontology lost one of their pioneers when Austin Brockenbrough Chinn, MD, died on November 25, 1989. A clinician, an investigator, an academic leader, and, above all, a creative organizer and advocate for improved health care for the elderly, Dr. Chinn inspired his colleagues and assisted at the rebirth of modern geriatrics. This book is dedicated to his memory.

Born in Warsaw, Virginia, he was educated at the University of Virginia and received his MD degree in 1932. After medical school, Dr. Chinn moved to Cleveland to train in internal medicine at University Hospitals of Cleveland. During this time he did research with Dr. Tom Spies, publishing six landmark papers on endemic pellagra. In Cleveland he also met his future wife, Ellen Wade, whom he married in 1938. After two years on the medical faculty at George Washington University, he entered practice in Washington, DC, before serving for four years as lieutenant colonel in the U.S. Army Medical Corps.

After World War II, Dr. Chinn was asked by Dean Joseph T. Wearn to return to Cleveland to join the rejuvenated medical faculty at Western Reserve University, where, during the following 16 years, he rose from assistant clinical professor to become associate professor and, eventually, associate dean. Dr. Chinn also practiced medicine during these years, and was one of the most admired internists and personal physicians in the community. His subsequent achievements, though frequently innovative, never failed to reflect his personal commitment to the welfare of the patient and the needs of practitioners in the field.

In 1952 Dr. Chinn accepted the position of medical director of the new Benjamin Rose Hospital (BRH), a unique inpatient facility built by the Benjamin Rose Institute, a philanthropic organization serving the elderly since 1908. (The new hospital was operated jointly with University Hospitals and the Department of Medicine of Western Reserve University School of Medicine.) During the next eight years Dr. Chinn's vision and effort brought into existence an original program for the comprehensive treatment and rehabilitation of chronic diseases of the aged. A multidisciplinary staff, consisting initially of only internists, was later supplemented by an orthopedist, a psychiatrist, and a rheumatologist. These medical specialists worked closely with strong departments of nursing, social work, and physical and occupational therapy to provide comprehensive care. The BRH staff was among the first to establish regular team case conferences as a means of analyzing geriatric cases in depth and developing multidisciplinary plans.

The hospital also became an educational center, with required rotations for house officers in medicine, acting internships for fourth-year medical students, and various assignments for students of nursing, social work, and physical therapy. Research laboratories had been included in the design of the hospital. Within the first 5 years a multilevel research program was under way, including basic research on the aging of collagen, other aspects of the pathology of aging, clinical studies of the outcome of treatment in arthritis, hip fracture, and stroke, and what is now known as health services research. In 1955 Dr. Chinn, with his director of social work, published a study describing quantitative, objective measurements of the course of physical disability in hospitalized old persons. Another member of the BRH staff, Sidney Katz, MD, strongly encouraged by Dr. Chinn, then went on to develop the now widely used Index of Activities of Daily Living. In 1960, Dr. Chinn received a 7-year grant from the National Institute on Aging (the largest such grant up to that time) for research in biological and behavioral aspects of aging.

Dr. Chinn's contact with federal officials in public health who shared his perception of the future importance of geriatrics led him, in 1960, to turn the direction of BRH over to a junior colleague in 1960 while he explored possibilities for wider application of his ideas as associate dean of Western Reserve School of Medicine.

Two years later he was called to Washington by the U.S. Public Health Service to direct the establishment of the Gerontology Branch of the Division of Chronic Services, where he served as chief of this new organization for four years. Building on his previous experience, he assembled a team of physicians, medical social workers, public health nurses, sociologists, program analysts, statisticians, writers, public health generalists, and management staff. Working also with the American Geriatrics Society, he molded his diverse group into a smoothly functioning organization. His goal was to develop "a curriculum in applied gerontology"—a goal that was realized by the publication of a four-volume series that he edited, entitled *Working with Older People: A Guide to Practice*. The final volume of this work evolved into a standard geriatric textbook, *Clinical Aspects of Aging*, now in its third edition (1989), under the editorship of William Reichel, MD.

Although he found government bureaucracy constantly frustrating, he won the respect of colleagues at all levels, insisting on close coordination between governmental and professional organizations. He eventually became a valued witness before the Senate in hearings related to the new Medicare law. He encouraged projects that made use of multiphasic health testing to foster health maintenance and preventive medicine among the elderly, and he initiated federal sponsorship of demonstration programs of adult day care, health counseling, information and referral, wellness clinics, and treatment programs for the elderly. The National Institute on Adult Daycare of the National Council on Aging survives as additional evidence of Dr. Chinn's initiative.

In the final phase of his professional career, Austin Chinn accepted the offer of a former colleague, Roger O. Egeberg, MD, then dean of the University of Southern California School of Medicine, to come to Los Angeles to help give emphasis, direction, and prestige to their new programs in geriatrics and rehabilitation. Dr. Egeberg recalls that, as professor of medicine and director of the Rehabilitation Research and Training Center, Dr. Chinn "organized and did a splendid job for the Medical School in setting up programs and forwarding the cause of rehabilitation medicine."

Austin Chinn was an exceptionally self-effacing man who valued family and privacy more than honors and the limelight. He retired quietly to his beloved Virginia in 1969. A colleague from the Washington days recalls, as do all of us who had the privilege of working with him, "his great intelligence, his impressive experience as a medical practitioner and as an academic leader, and his extraordinary decency and integrity." Another friend adds to this, describing Dr. Chinn as: "modest, reserved, strong sense of justice, serious turn of mind, sparked occasionally with wry humor, compassionate and caring. He was an idealist with vision." Geriatric medicine and gerontology acknowledges a great debt to this remarkable man.

AMASA B. FORD, MD

Preface

The daily stresses and strains that affect the health of older adults have only recently come into focus. Identification of such stressors is becoming a significant part of research pertaining to elders. Management of stress plays a critical role in the lives of aged persons and often affects their quality of life and health status. New perspectives on various sources of stress, strategies for diagnosis and treatment, and responses of older adults to stress were highlighted during the 10th Annual Symposium hosted by the University Center on Aging and Health and the Geriatric Education Center of CWRU. This timely conference on stress and health among the elderly was held in October 1990 and was attended by 200 doctors, nurses, psychologists, and social workers from across the country. This book grew out of the presentations and discussions at the conference.

There are several goals for this book. The first is to educate health professionals regarding the interaction of stress and health based on information from research. The second goal is to review theories on stress and health, and their application to elderly persons. Another goal is to analyze the impact of extreme stress, cumulative stress, and chronic stress on older adults, and to describe the types of behavioral and immunological responses of elderly persons to stress. A fourth goal is to examine the racial and ethical aspects that influence stress and health in aged persons, and to assess the elderly person's use of protective mechanisms including individual coping, and social and family supports. Current psychotherapeutic interventions and pharmacological treatment used for stress in the elderly are also addressed. Finally, because of the need for more research concerning stress and health among older adults, a section is devoted to the exploration of conceptual and measurement issues in stress research.

With the expected increase in the number of aged adults and with concerns about the mental health and mental health treatment of this aged group, it is imperative that health professionals become more astute in their approach to those older persons experiencing stress. In the past, it was believed that elderly persons did not benefit from systematic strategies and interventions to reduce stress. Using an interdisciplinary approach, however, we are finding that older adults do respond favorably to treatment and can learn new coping strategies to reduce their stress.

This book, divided into three parts, addresses the problems of comprehensive assessment and treatment of stress in older adults and the effect of stress on their health. The first part presents an overview of stress and health issues among elderly persons, and examines several theoretical frameworks for coping. The section also examines the social support process. The second section describes the health and functioning of the elderly related to loss as well as a study of widowhood, the adaptation of aged persons to extreme stress, and a focus on the critical issues regarding stress and health among the minority aged. The last section discusses various treatment measures used for older persons who are stressed, and examines stress experiences related to different environments of care and immune response. The book closes with an epilogue by Eva Kahana, Pierce T. and Elizabeth Robson Professor of Humanities, CWRU. She provides a thought-provoking synopsis of the salient points presented by the contributors. Dr. Eva Kahana challenges researchers to move beyond life events as discrete stressors and consider stress experienced by older adults as events reflecting environmental stress as well as the effects of exposure to earlier stressors on late life adaptation. It is hoped that this book will highlight some of the controversies surrounding the care issues of older persons exposed to stress because stress has an impact on the entire society as well as the individual and family. We wish to recognize the following persons for their help in preparation for this manuscript: Beth Kaskel, Tsui Chan, Subhash Sharma, Sanjay Menon, Ajay Dass, Christine Cunningham, Dean Handy, and Karen Tecco. We also wish to thank Diane Ferris for her help in producing both the conference and this book.

PART I
Elements of Stress Model: Focus on Theory and Method

The stress paradigm embodies within it some of the most exciting and challenging aspects of social science research relevant to psychosocial well-being. Research that has used the stress paradigm for understanding well-being of the aged has revealed the attractiveness, complexities, and ambiguities of the paradigm. Chapters in this section explore understandings that have been gained through applying conceptual and methodological advances in the field of stress research to issues facing the elderly.

Social scientists seeking to discern meaningful patterns in complex social phenomena must develop special skills. They must be able to note regularities in behaviors and experiences of individuals in the context of the rich fabric of society and develop theoretical models that explain such regularities. To do so, they must be able to distinguish forests from trees; note key relationships amid multitudes of variables; and even as they build cogent and parsimonious models, they must remember that at best they have succeeded in understanding one small corner in the vast world of social phenomena.

The focus of Kasl's overview chapter is on the independent variable of stress and the outcome variable of health within the stress paradigm. Kasl presents an extensive overview and thorough critique of the classical and contemporary theoretical literature surrounding the concept of stress in a psychosocial context, focusing on methodological considerations. He also provides illuminating results from a Yale University study on the epidemiology of health and aging. He concludes in his overview of stress and health among the elderly that the impact of psychosocial factors on health status is not dramatically altered by age.

Chiriboga's emphasis is also on the independent variable of stress among components of the stress paradigm. Chiriboga provides a historical overview of directions in the study of stress, ranging from catastrophic models to life event stress and stressors of everyday life. Chiriboga uses his own studies of stress in middle and late life to illustrate challenges of operationalizing and measuring diverse concepts of stress. He contends that the measurement approaches used today need to be reassessed, and new instrumentation needs to be developed to assess particular stress conditions more in-depth. At the same time, he acknowledges that proliferations of assessment tools pose problems in achieving comparability among studies using different assessment strategies.

The chapters by Jackson and Antonucci, and by Aldwin focus on resources that buffer the adverse effects of stress. Jackson and Antonucci highlight social support, the major external resource that has been studied as a buffer of stress, whereas the focus of Aldwin's treatise is on internal resources of coping and efficacy, which are major internal resources in the context of the stress paradigm.

Jackson and Antonucci's chapter provides a thorough review of the social support literature from 1947 to the present. The authors note that classical definitions of social support lack a clear focus and confuse issues of social integration with social networks, ties, and evaluations.

Recent literature attempts to explain socially supportive relationships and their consequences on individuals and families using a life-course framework. The authors conclude that social support needs to be conceptualized and researched within a life-span or life-course theoretical framework. They, too, discuss the issue of measurement and suggest that multidimensional and longitudinal studies are needed for operationalizing other more comprehensive understandings of social support processes.

Aldwin's discussion of coping and efficacy in a life-span developmental context presents an interesting counterpoint to Kasl's view about the lack of relevance of age to the stress paradigm. Aldwin argues that a study of age-specific aspects of coping in fact allows for a better understanding of adult development and aging. Her discussion reviews age differences in stress and coping processes as well as the life-span developmental approach related to the stress process. Her arguments are illustrated by presentation of two empirical studies of coping that evolved from the life-span theoretical framework. Finally, she directs the research community to develop age-sensitive instruments that will permit assessment of developmental changes in the coping process.

Each of the four contributors in this section takes a broad and comprehensive view of the stress process even as the authors focus on different components of the stress paradigm. The relevance of age to understanding of the stress process is also addressed in each chapter. Each author seeks to understand the stress paradigm in a relatively comprehensive manner. In doing so, they invoke the historical, theoretical, and methodological contexts within which stress research is embedded. The "big picture" of stress research and the generalizations it permits, which are explored in the first section of the book, pave the way for consideration of diversity in response to stress considered in subsequent chapters.

The contributions in this section well illustrate the rapid progress being made in stress research relevant to the elderly. Each contribution provides a valuable glimpse into the value of alternative conceptual orientations and methodological approaches in the field of stress research and delineates directions that can lead to applying what has been learned to practice and policy in gerontology.

1

Stress and Health Among the Elderly: Overview of Issues

Stanislav V. Kasl

The high marquee value of the concept of "stress" is exceeded only by the amount of scientific and linguistic controversy that surrounds it. Thus a presentation of issues concerning stress and health of the elderly must begin with some attempts to charter this territory of ambiguous boundaries, and to provide some rational organization to the themes and issues. A serviceable overview of this topic needs to inform in a neutral fashion, without exacerbating old controversies or creating new ones. Unfortunately, given the long history of dissension and confusion, advocating even such apparently "reasonable" positions as that of abandonment of the concept of stress, or that of the absolute need for uniformity of conceptual and linguistic usage represents a controversial remedy that will feed the acrimony rather than provide an acceptable solution.

It is my personal observation that stress anthologies (or conferences or workshops or seminars) that aim to straighten out the mess, reach clarity and consensus, and provide guidelines for the future actually accomplish very little. This leads me to two conclusions. First, a tolerant pluralism regarding stress formulations and approaches is at present a practical necessity. Second, a heavy reliance on "stress" as a central concept, as an organizing formulation that guides hypotheses, operationalizations, and interpretations, is not as wise a course of action as using "stress" as a minor crutch, a concept that has a lot of surplus meaning and rich connotations, but that is replaced with more specific and precise conceptualizations as soon as one is discussing the particulars of a research domain.

Above all, it is important to realize that, whatever one's approach and whatever one's terminology, there is an absolute need for clarity in communication. Specifically, the reader and the audience must always be in a position to translate *stress*, when the word is used, into the actual operationalizations that were used and the actual data that were collected.

Given the preceding comments, it would seem that the goals of this book can be stated broadly (and quite ambitiously) as follows: We wish to examine the role of stress in the etiology of disease and the etiology of health status changes among the elderly. The term "stress" represents an incomplete and open-ended specification of a variety of social and psychological factors and exposures (experiences) that may influence the health of the elderly. It is far better to be inclusive so that we may have a comprehensive picture of the psychosocial influences on the health status of the elderly than to agonize over whether a particular risk factor is properly grouped among a class of risk factors called stress, and thus become exclusive and narrow because of a particular usage of the term stress.

The fact that we are concentrating on the health of the *elderly* does not mean that we should ignore other segments of the population. Properly, we need to adopt a *comparative* approach: *How* does the etiological picture for stress and disease vary by age of persons studied, and *why* is there such a variation in etiological dynamics?

Of course, such a broad statement of goals for this book will remain only an unattainable ideal. Not only is our understanding of the role of psychosocial risk factors in the etiology of disease quite fragmentary, but sound comparisons across stages of the life cycle and generations are truly impossible in most instances.

CONCEPT OF STRESS IN CONTEXT OF PSYCHOSOCIAL EPIDEMIOLOGY

Clearly, the term stress continues to be used in several fundamentally different ways. This is true both when it is used loosely and informally in the vernacular as well as when it is formally defined and embedded in a formal theoretical structure or a formal program of research. The categories of usage are as follows:

1. Stress as a *stimulus* condition that is objectively defined or susceptible to objective measurement. Approximate synonyms for stimulus condition are independent variable, risk factor, and exposure variable. The term *objective* is, of course, somewhat slippery, but the general idea is to designate measurement that does not intentionally involve the subject's cognitive and emotional processing (see Frese & Zapf, 1988).

2. Stress as an *appraisal* of an environmental condition or of an experience. This is still a stimulus approach to stress, but it is a psychological or subjective orientation. A strong version of this approach asserts that the subjective appraisal is the unique and sole mediating process between the objective stimulus and the health outcome.

3. Stress as a *response* to the environmental condition or to its appraisal.

4. Stress as a complex *relational* or *interactive* term, linking the environmental demands and the person's capacity to meet the demands. In such a complex, relational term, the logical possibility exists of using purely objective variables, purely subjective ones, or some mixture of the two.

The multiplicity of usages is not, by any means, all of the problem. In addition, we lack agreement (and we lack compelling guidelines on how to develop agreement) on defining criteria, on *criterial properties* of stress. Suppose, for example, consensus was reached that stress should be used only as an objective stimulus condition. We still do not have agreed-on a priori conceptual criteria for the existence of a stressor. What we do have are intuitive lists of exemplary concrete experiences or exposures we propose as stressors, plus some vague general notion of "excessive" environmental demands. Similarly, we might achieve consensus that "stress" should be used as a response. Is there a unique stress reaction, however, and which parameters—biomedical, psychological, or behavioral—define it? Do we wish to commit ourselves to the notion that a certain kind of reactivity, measured by specified parameters, defines stress, its presence, or its absence?

A good illustration of the linguistic and conceptual morass that is occasionally engendered in the stress field can be seen in the attempts to distinguish between "good" stress and "bad" stress, as in Selye's (1983) writings on "eustress" and "understress." The idea here, fundamentally, is to postulate an optimal level of stress so that either too little or too much is presumed to be pathogenic. This idea would be reasonable only if one wished to equate stress with such concepts as arousal, activation, stimulation, or challenge. Few in the field, however, would be comfortable with such an equivalence. Thus it is awkward to have some equate stress with challenge, whereas many others equate stress with the conviction that the challenge cannot be met (i.e., an "excessive" challenge). Also, those who use the response meaning of stress, such as equating "stress" with symptoms of distress or tension or dysphoria, would encounter difficulty with the notion of "good" stress. This kind of a morass may likely be self-inflicted. Why not simply deal with certain specific concepts as independent variables (e.g., deadline pressures or job insecurity) and with other specific concepts as dependent variables (e.g., quality of work, absenteeism, depression, or heart disease), and then try to establish the nature of the functional relationship between the two, whether it be linear, threshold, or curvilinear?

The absence of consensus on criterial properties of stress—whether used as a stimulus condition or as a response—creates problems of defining the *scope* and *boundaries* in a review chapter on stress and health. Consider, for example, the currently popular concept of *social support* and its influence on health (e.g., Berkman, 1984; Cohen, 1988; Cohen & Syme, 1985; Sarason & Sarason, 1985; Shumaker & Czajkowski, in press). It has become fully de rigueur to treat social support and stress as completely distinct concepts, albeit examined frequently for their joint or interactive influence on health. There is nothing about the notions of social isolation, lack of a confidant, or an unsupportive spouse, however, that could not be encompassed in most formulations of the stress concept. In fact, the potential for conceptual overlap between the two constructs is substantial. For example, in the Cohen and Syme (1985) book, social support is defined as "the resources provided by other persons" (p. 4). Stress, conversely, is generically seen as some imbalance between environmental demands and response capability (e.g., McGrath, 1970). Because resource by definition enhances response capability, the conceptual linkage between stress and social support borders on redundancy.

Another currently popular broad concept is that of *control*. Within the wide domain of psychosocial epidemiology, it has become prominent in such areas as aging (e.g., Rodin, 1986; Rodin, Timko, & Harris, 1985) and occupational epidemiology (e.g., Sauter, Hurrell, & Cooper, 1989). An appropriate definition of control, which encompasses most of the notions about control that have been proposed, would be in terms of "control as some response availability to influence, in an intended direction, an important outcome" (Kasl, 1989, p. 164). Once again, however, the conceptual overlap with stress (and social support as well) is considerable. Incidentally, the literature on control generally makes the distinction between perception of control and "actual" control; this, too, fully parallels stress theory—that is, the distinction between objective and subjective aspects of the stimulus condition.

Some appreciation of the difficulties of trying to work with stress as a scientific construct, and as a risk factor for disease, is to pose an apparently simple, and an apparently appropriate, question: Is stress among the elderly greater than among younger adults? It is difficult to see how we should go about tackling this question. Suppose we answer: No, stress is less among the elderly because data using summative scales of stressful life events show that the elderly report considerably fewer life events (e.g., Goldberg & Comstock, 1980; Masuda & Holmes, 1978). It is safe to assume that such an answer would be met with severe criticism. One sure form of criticism would be to point out that a single measure, a single operationalization, cannot possibly encompass the full meaning of such a broad construct. Those who endorse the stimulus approach to stress would point to the need to include other stress exposures with measures reflecting hassles, small life events, and chronic stressful situations (for more detail on these concepts and measures, see Chiriboga, 1989). Agreement on specific choices of measurement procedures might not be high, and developing strategies for combining information from these disparate measures might be difficult. Those who approach the concept of stress from the response side would presumably object equally strongly to the notion that a single measure could reflect this broad concept. Consensus on what responses to measure, however, would seem to be less likely here than for the stimulus side of stress. The strategy of a mix of measures such as self-report, behavioral performance, psychophysiological, neuroendocrine (e.g., Baum, Grunberg, & Singer, 1982) appears attractive at first glance. In fact, however, these are best seen as indicators of reactivity obtained in a setting of acute exposure and needing some form of before and after measurement for proper interpretation. Their sensitivity and appropriateness for reflecting the impact of longer-lasting exposures in a real-life setting, with a single measurement, are likely to be quite limited. Various symptom-based indicators of anxiety, tension, distress, or dysphoric mood offer another possible approach to measuring stress levels. It is difficult to see, however, why the influence of stable personality traits, such as neuroticism, does not constitute a major source of contamination that seriously threatens the usefulness of these measures for such a purpose (see Costa & McCrae, 1989). It would also seem to be highly controversial to attempt to select specific diagnostic categories as indicators of stress, such as alcohol abuse, ulcers, inflammatory bowel syndrome, and so on. The notion that certain disorders could be designated as "stress disorders" goes strongly against the recognition that such disorders invariably have multiple etiology or multiple risk factors. Finally, one might adopt a strategy of using measures that reflect a direct appraisal of stress, such as the Perceived Stress Scale (Cohen, 1986; Cohen, Kamarck, & Mermelstein, 1983). Items on this scale are intended to reflect how unpredictable, uncontrollable, and overloading respondents find their lives; this approach is the most direct operationalization of a global, subjectivist approach to stress. Unfortunately, although the scale does intend to measure the respondent's appraisal of life circumstances, it remains difficult not to judge this scale as another response-based measure of stress, though perhaps existing measures of nonspecific psychological distress, such as demoralization (Dohrenwend, Shrout, Egri, & Mendelsohn, 1980), will not completely account for its variance.

We gain further insight into the difficulties of coordinating the concept of stress to a particular operationalization or set of operationalizations if we focus in on a single approach, the summative stressful life events scale, as exemplified by the oldest one, the Holmes and Rahe (1967) Social Readjustment Rating Scale (SRRS). Several investigators (e.g., George, 1980; Murrell, Norris, & Hutchins, 1984) have modified the original SRE instrument by including new items that reflect the life events likely to be experienced in later life. Although such modifications appear to reviewers (e.g., Chiriboga, 1989) to be a most reasonable modification of the instrument, in fact they do raise some questions. For one, if items are added for the explicit reason that the elderly are more likely to report such events, then can we still use such instruments to compare stress levels across age groups? The answer would seem to be "no." Furthermore, on what basis should specific events be added, or not added? The answer is not clear. Are events added because they impact on health and well-being, because they are transitions known to create readjustment demands, or because they reflect someone's intuitive notion of "change" in the daily life of the elderly? The fact that one instrument (Amster & Krauss, 1974) included "reaching the age of 65" as an item suggests the potential absurdity of some of the additional items. In fact, it must be concluded that such instruments may remain quite reasonable as indicators of a specified (or specifiable, or unspecified) domain of life events or changes, but they become less satisfactory as operationalizations of stress.

It is possible to make this point quite general. Each candidate measure of stress has a dual role. First, it measures what it measures. That is, it has specific content that needs to be stated precisely and narrowly (e.g., working 20 hours overtime, reporting to two bosses, placing one's spouse in a nursing home, reporting symptoms of tension, having high serum cortisol levels, etc.). Second, it measures stress. The latter presupposes that there is an adequate theory specifying the nature of this construct so that one could evaluate the adequacy of a particular measure as a partial operationalization of this construct. To the extent that the concept of stress is not embedded in a well-specified theory and network of other constructs—and I believe that such a situation does not exist as yet—then it is prudent to fall back on the first role of these candidate measures and refer to them in the narrow and specific terms only.

From the perspective of history of science, it is interesting to speculate on the rise and fall of major broad constructs that have dominated the general domain of social science and medicine (including psychosocial epidemiology)—that is, such concepts as stress, social support, and control. In the early stages, they reflect the need for overarching constructs that will bring diverse phenomena and ideas together, and will generate new hypotheses and interpretations of findings. In the process, however, such constructs may become too broad, imprecise, unmanageable. Thus, when one begins to try to integrate the accumulated evidence and, particularly, when one begins to search for mechanisms and mediating processes, one feels compelled to deal with specific risk factors and specific outcomes, and the broad concept begins to fractionate and recede in usefulness. With respect to stress, the present situation is difficult to diagnose. At what stage of this cycle is the concept, and has it gone through several such cycles already? Most likely, different investigators in the stress field would give rather different responses, which may be still another dimension of disagreement, thus contributing to the general feeling that one can neither live with the concept nor without it.

SOME METHODOLOGICAL CONSIDERATIONS IN STUDYING STRESS AND HEALTH AMONG THE ELDERLY

Aging, Stress, and Health (Markides & Cooper, 1989) provides a good glimpse of the different research content areas that, collectively, can serve to characterize the research domain to be considered briefly in this section from a methodological perspective. Most stress and health studies on the elderly seem to fall into the following three categories:

1. The first group is investigations of the impact of specific life events or experiences. The prototypic studies in this group have dealt with retirement, bereavement (widowhood), institutionalization, and relocation or residential change. Studies of natural disasters and traumas would also fall in here, but they are not very common.

2. The second group of studies uses as its basic instrument a summative stressful life events scale, generally the Holmes and Rahe (1967) SRRS or some modification of it. Although these studies, like those in the first group, appear to converge on the stimulus side of stress and emphasize the experience of change in one's life circumstances, the typical methodology of these two sets of studies sets them clearly apart. There are other instrument-driven studies in which the orienting concept is hassles rather than life events (e.g., Kanner, Coyne, Schaefer, & Lazarus, 1981). They have been classified as "stressor of the micro level" (Chiriboga, 1989), but it is not clear whether they should be seen primarily as minor life events, or if they should be classified with response-based approaches to stress because of their emphasis on the reactions (e.g., irritation, frustration, and distress) the respondents report that they caused.

3. The third group of studies deals with chronic or enduring socio-environmental stressors. In the total stress field, many of the studies deal with occupational stress, but of course very little of it is on the

elderly. The literature on family stress—that is, parent-child or hus-band-wife relations—also tends to exclude the elderly. Conversely, studies of caregiver burden (e.g., Montgomery, 1989) tend to concentrate on the elderly. Other content areas that fall in here would be studies of the residential environment, social isolation–social relationship, and (to a small extent) financial stressors.

The methodological concerns that arise in studies of stress and health in the elderly will be outlined as being linked either to the measurement of stress or to the general design of the study (including choice of data analysis strategies). Because such studies are seeking to describe the health impact of stress, the formulation of methodological concerns will often be in terms of threats to the validity of such a causal interpretation and in terms of alternative explanations. This is the strategy so well developed by Cook and Campbell (1979).

With respect to the summative stressful life-events approach, content of the scale items has already been raised as a difficulty. In addition, there would seem to be three major concerns:

1. *Self-selection into events (experiences)*: Individuals do not experience events in a random fashion; rather life events are embedded in social structures, in life-style and life-cycle characteristics, and these may be the variables of underlying etiological significance, or the variables whose influence must be partialed out. For example, Masuda and Holmes (1978) have reported on the annual frequencies of life events and have shown that heroin addicts and alcoholics experience about 5 times as many events as medical students, football players, and pregnant mothers. This suggests that, for example, addicts and alcoholics have life-styles that precipitate high rates of life events; it is unlikely, however, that individuals who at some point are exposed to many life events are at increased risk of later becoming addicts and alcoholics.

2. *Confounding of independent and dependent variables*: Many items on the list of events are, in fact, indicators of health and functioning, the very variables that are the studied outcomes.

3. *Biased reporting of events*: Many of the events on these lists represent vague or ambiguous, partially subjective, experiences. Thus aside from potential biases resulting from memory, there may be strong individual differences in threshold of recognition that an event does apply and in threshold of willingness to report the (mostly

negative) events. Respondents' current health status, or mood and affect, may influence the reporting of events, as much the search for meaning among cases with a particular disease under study. These methodological points are discussed at greater length elsewhere (Kasl, 1983, 1984b).

Strong designs can overcome some limitations of measurement but not all. Suppose we are dealing with a prospective study of stroke incidence among the elderly. If the number of reported stressful life events is found to predict stroke, net of other covariates such as age, hypertension, smoking, alcohol consumption, and so on, then it is likely that we are dealing with a variable, or an indicator of a variable, that is of etiological significance. Strictly speaking, however, we have only dealt with two problems: We have ruled out reverse causation (influence of disease on measured life events) and the confounding statistical influence of selected other variables. The proper interpretation of the etiological variable may remain elusive, however; influences on reporting of stressful life events, such as neuroticism or negative affectivity (Watson & Pennebaker, 1989), could be involved, as could some underlying self-selection factor. In weak designs, such as retrospective case-control studies, it is difficult to rule out any of the potential threats to validity. It is significant to note that the apparently impressive evidence on stressful life events and health outcomes is based on weak designs, and prospective studies that use careful statistical adjustments of relevant covariates tend to yield negative results (Kasl, 1984a).

The summative stressful life events approach represents premature closure on a hypothesis that still needs testing—that is, that life events, regardless of desirability, create readjustment demands that summate in impact (regardless of the specific combination of items) and increase generalized susceptibility to illness in a dose-response fashion. Thus, studies that examine the impact of a *single* life event, such as retirement or widowhood, have many potential research design advantages. For example, one can schedule data collection at specific times after exposure to check on stages of impact, adaptation, and recovery. Alternatively, one can include moderator variables that condition the impact of a specific life event. Because one is focusing on a single event, one generally has objective information that the exposure did occur, and one may even have additional information on differential characteristics of the exposure for subgroups of individuals.

Several research design considerations come into play when one is focusing on the impact of a single life event. Two of the most important issues are closely linked to each other: availability of baseline (or preexposure) data and self-selection factors. In general, events that are planned and predictable, such as retirement or a residential move to a retirement community, make it relatively easy to schedule preexposure data collection. At the same time, the planned nature of such changes makes it difficult to know when it is optimal to schedule the initial data collection. Just shortly before the change is likely to be a stage of anticipation and preparation, if not turmoil. Much longer before the change poses logistic difficulties and increases threat of attrition during follow-up. In fact, a change such as retirement is so fully anticipated (in the life-cycle sense) that preretirement planning and anticipation may become a highly variable characteristic of the respondents. Thus, selecting any one particular temporal distance from the event as the time of the first contact may do very little to guarantee comparable "baseline" data for all.

Events that are anticipated and planned are likely to represent a strong potential for the confounding role of self-selection variables. Thus, for example, in examining the impact of a move to a retirement community (Kasl & Rosenfield, 1980), it becomes difficult to disentangle the role of plans and intentions (including preferences not to move and desires to move that cannot be implemented) and reasons for the move from the impact of the change itself. Conversely, events that are truly unanticipated, such as natural disasters, do not allow scheduling of baseline data, unless one happens to be in the midst of a multiwave study set up for other reasons (Phifer, Kaniasty, & Norris, 1988). At the same time, however, the potential for self-selection bias in such disasters is generally low and may be limited to sociodemographic and residential characteristics.

Self-selection issues are salient when one is designing a study in which the elderly experiencing an event are compared with those who do not. The study of some events may be hampered by our inability to create reasonably comparable groups so that baseline inequalities can then be handled statistically. Thus, comparing elderly who are institutionalized with a community sample (Tobin & Lieberman, 1976) or early retirees with those who work past normal retirement age (Kasl, 1980) creates such substantial differences in baseline health status that statistical adjustments are likely to be unfeasible. It should also be noted that when strong selection bias operates on the variable on which the subjects are also followed for impact, such as health status, it is quite likely that baseline differences alone may not reflect all of the self-selection bias; that is, for example, just recently institutionalized elderly may be about to embark on a trajectory of health status decline that is likely to be steeper than for community controls, but close matching on initial health status will not adequately control for this difference.

The existence of self-selection factors may be underestimated in situations in which the event is precipitated by characteristics of others rather than the subject. Thus in bereavement, the death of a spouse is predictable from health status and other characteristics of the deceased, not the widowed person who is followed for impact. The fact that analyses of mortality after bereavement (Bowling, 1987), compared with those who continue to be married, generally do not (and are not able to) adjust for baseline health, thus, does not seem too bothersome. In fact, however, spousal similarity in important health habits such as smoking and important risk factors such as blood pressure may be considerable (e.g., Speers, Kasl, Freeman, & Ostfeld, 1986). Therefore the widowed, compared with the married, may be selected indirectly for higher risk of death.

Investigations of stress and health in the elderly in which the focus is on *chronic* or *enduring* socioenvironmental conditions, rather than change, raise the potential for serious methodological concerns whenever the measurement of the stressor involves subjective appraisal. These concerns are confounding, triviality, circularity, and interpretive muddle. As with summative stressful life-events scales, the issues are altered by variations in design and by type of dependent variable. Thus, if we are linking retrospective subjective accounts of exposure to outcomes (e.g., levels of distress), at time of interview, then there is a strong possibility of distress influencing the account. If there is a temporal separation between earlier subjective accounts of exposure and later measures of distress, we may be only measuring the temporal stability of some broad construct of "psychological reaction" to the exposure and its earlier versus later manifestations. If we are using evaluations and perceptions that are solidly anchored in stable predispositions (e.g., "How much control did you feel you had over the situation?"), then associations with outcome may be due to the role of this third variable rather than differences in the way the event appears to be appraised.

The strategy of using "objective" measures of stressors is central to attempts to reduce many of these methodological concerns. A more detailed reasoning for advocating this strategy can be found elsewhere (Kasl, 1985). Two additional comments are in order, however. One is that this strategy does not imply that objective measurement deals only with physical reality. For example, workers can be informed about their exposure to toxic materials (Houts & McDougall, 1988) and the act of informing them is susceptible to objective measurement; however, what is studied is not exposure to toxic substances (the physical reality) but exposure to information (the "symbolic" reality). The second point is that by emphasizing objective measurement approaches one is not necessarily ignoring the possibility that an objectively defined exposure may have different "meanings" to different individuals. Rather, what is being proposed is that this possibility of a variety of meanings should not automatically lead to an exclusive reliance on subjective appraisals and reactions. The challenge to investigators is to use variables that are relevant to individual differences in "meaning" of the exposure but are not direct measures of emotional processing. Ultimately, the argument is that a variety of measures are available to the investigators. They can be ordered as follows: (a) objective measures of exposure; (b) additional objective characteristics of the situation and individuals exposed, so that subtypes of exposures can be generated; (c) objective characteristics of individuals that may be moderator variables; (d) measures of traits and dispositions, also potential moderators; (e) self-reports of exposure, devoid of evaluations and reactions; (f) evaluations and appraisals of exposure; and (g) affective reactions to exposure (e.g., bothered, concerned, or distressed). The basic point is that exclusive reliance on the last two types of measures is undesirable and creates many methodological problems.

The final methodological point to be discussed concerns the strategy of using longitudinal designs in studies of stress and health in the elderly. There is no doubt that most investigators appreciate many or most of the limitations of cross-sectional data. Many of these investigators also believe that whatever is wrong with cross-sectional data can be fixed with longitudinal data. The point to be developed here is that the virtues of longitudinal designs have been overestimated.

To begin with, it is useful to distinguish among three types of longitudinal designs. (a) *Doubly prospective:* The cohort is picked up

before exposure to the risk factor (stressful event or stressful environmental condition) and before development of the target disease. (b)
Prospective: The cohort is free of target disease but exposure to the risk
factor has already occurred (among those who will be classified as
exposed). (c) Merely longitudinal ("slice of life"): We have a cross-
sectional picture of elderly people's lives at an arbitrary (random)
point in their life cycle and then we recontact them one or more times
at evenly spaced (but arbitrary) intervals to create a "window" on
their lives. It is this third type of longitudinal design that is commonest in social gerontology and psychosocial epidemiology of the aging;
typically, one has a sample of community living elderly, 65 and older,
who are followed with additional interviews and monitored for selected outcomes. Well-established data analysis strategies use baseline
data as predictors or covariates in examining status at some later time.
It is this third type of longitudinal design, the virtues of which have
been exaggerated.

It is possible to make several interrelated points about the slice-of-
life design. One is that if the cohort is in a steady state (i.e., nothing
much is happening), then longitudinal analysis is not likely to improve on the interpretability of cross-sectional associations. Lagged
correlations will reflect temporal stability and will not hint at likely
causal priorities. Predicting change, net of baseline status, may be
futile because changes may mostly reflect measurement error.

A second related point may be labeled "left censoring." In this case,
we generally have no information (except for historical records or
retrospection) about earlier states of the cohort with respect to the
putative risk factor and outcome. Suppose, for example, that having
very small social networks increases the risk of adverse health status
changes. Baseline cross-sectional association in the expected direction
will not be conclusive; poor health could lead to small networks. If
the effect of network size has already played itself out during the
10 years before the cohort was picked up, then no further health
deficits will be observed in longitudinal analysis because the cohort
was picked up too late for that phenomenon to be detected. If the
effect has not yet played itself out, then the risk associated with small
networks will be detected even if the cohort appears to be in a steady
state with respect to the independent variable. Conversely, the benefits of an increase in size of network will not be detected if the effects
of the previous state are cumulative and delayed.

A third point is that even in the absence of a steady state, temporal ordering of variables may not be established in the slice-of-life design. For example, in a 4-year follow-up of a sample of Chicago residents (Pearlin, Lieberman, Menaghan, & Mullan, 1981), data were collected on disruptions of work life (e.g., fired, laid off, downgraded, or left work because of illness) for the interim 4-year interval; a complex analysis of the results led to the interpretation that such disruptions contributed to diminished self-concept (e.g., self-esteem or mastery) and higher depression. It does not seem likely, however, that even a highly sophisticated statistical treatment of initial values of self-esteem or depression (covariates) can satisfactorily dispose of the alternative hypothesis that (unmeasured) adverse changes in self-esteem or depression preceded many of the disruptions in work life. The logistically awkward solution here is to have sufficiently frequent contacts with the cohort so that the temporal separation of the variables of interests, if it exists, can be detected.

SOME ILLUSTRATIVE FINDINGS FROM YALE'S EPIDEMIOLOGY OF AGING PROGRAM

In this section I wish to offer selected findings from the ongoing research program on the epidemiology of aging in Yale's Department of Epidemiology and Public Health. These findings are intended to reflect some of the points that have been made in the previous pages as well as to illustrate the possible promise of psychosocial variables that may influence the health of the elderly but are not conventionally considered under the label stress.

First, we shall present some data on the impact of bereavement. The results are based on data collected in the Yale Health and Aging Project, which is part of the National Institute on Aging–funded Established Populations for Epidemiologic Studies of the Elderly (EPESE) Program (Cornoni-Huntley, Brock, Ostfeld, Taylor, & Wallace, 1986). The Yale component involves some 2,812 noninstitutionalized community-living elderly (65 and older) who were sampled by three housing strata: public elderly housing, private elderly housing, and a general community stratum. The cohort was interviewed in the home in 1982, and again in 1985 and 1988. Briefer telephone interviews were conducted yearly in the other years. The cohort was monitored for mortality, hospitalizations, and nursing home placements. Greater detail on the methodology is given in Berkman et al. (1986).

Complete monitoring of the cohort (and their spouses) has allowed us to look at short-term mortality after bereavement (Mendes de Leon, Kasl, & Jacobs, 1991). The analysis differs in two important ways from previous studies. First, it examines the effect in a cohort of married persons by using a proportional hazards model with time-dependent covariates for onset of widowhood and time since widowhood rather than retroactively matching the widowed with subjects remaining married throughout follow-up. Second, detailed information was available on prewidowhood health status and other risk factors, which permitted rigorous control for health status inequalities between the married and widowed. Data analysis was based on the 1,046 married subjects at baseline. During follow-up of about 7 years, 103 men and 136 women became widowed. Analyses were done for young-old (younger than 74 years) and old-old women separately, as mortality risks among recent widows varied significantly by age. Younger widows had relative risks (RR) of 3.11 and 2.20 during the first 6 and 12 months after widowhood, which increased in magnitude after adjustment for socioeconomic status, risk behaviors, and health status. Excess risk among older widows was not observed. Widowers had significant crude RRs of 2.67 and 2.25 for 6 and 12 months, but these decreased to nonsignificant levels after adjustment. These findings suggest that previously observed elevated risks among widowers and weaker risks among widows may have been affected by inadequate gender-specific adjustments of prewidowhood health status.

In Table 1.1, we present some preliminary data on depression and bereavement; the scale used is the CESD (Radloff, 1977). Several findings are noteworthy. (a) At baseline (1982), the respondents who later become bereaved are already significantly higher on depression than respondents who remain married through the 1982–85 follow-up. This suggests an impact of the (presumably) poor health of the spouse who later dies. (b) The change data show a significant impact of the bereavement experience; further analyses (gender by age by bereaved status interaction) reveal a lack of impact among the older widowed women. (c) The bottom of the table reveals that an impact on depression is primarily seen among those who become widowed within a year of the follow-up interview. This is presumably a function of two effects: the impact of bereavement is self-limited, and the

TABLE 1.1 Depression Before and After Spousal Bereavement

		Men		Women	
		65–74	75+	65–74	75+
Mean depression (CESD)	Still married	5.2	7.0	7.9	10.3
at baseline (1982)	Bereaved	7.8	8.0	8.6	11.6
Mean 3-year change in	Still Married	0.6	0.3	0.6	2.1
depression (1985 minus 1982)	Bereaved	2.9	3.2	5.2	−0.6
Mean 3-year change in depression, bereaved only	Death within 2 years of 1982 interview	−2.9	1.2	2.8	−3.8
	Death within 1 year of 1985 interview	8.0	9.8	9.6	6.4

prebereavement elevation (seen in point a) is less likely because the 1982 interview was at least 2 years before the spousal death. This links up to the previous discussion of the slice-of-life longitudinal design: the frequency of data collection on the cohort is important, as is the temporal location of a particular stressful event in relation to the "before" and "after" data collection points. In a longitudinal survey of older adults in which the cohort was interviewed at 6-month intervals (Murrell & Himmelfarb, 1989), it was much more clearly apparent that by 1 year postbereavement, most of the impact on depression is gone. This is fully consistent with results from another study of bereavement (Kasl, Ostfeld, Berkman, & Jacobs, 1987) where depression data were available at 6 weeks, 6 months, 1 year, and 2 years after bereavement. Incidentally, this study showed no impact of bereavement on alcohol consumption.

The Yale community survey of 2,812 elderly contains data on some 330 spouse pairs—that is, when both spouses are part of the study. This lends itself to an analysis in which the health and functioning of one spouse are examined for their impact on the other spouse. One type of such analysis concerned itself with the impact of mild and moderate levels of cognitive impairment, as measured by the SPMSQ (Pfeiffer, 1975), on the health and well-being of the other spouse (Moritz, 1987; Moritz, Kasl, & Berkman, 1989). The major findings are highlighted in Table 1.2 and represent results of cross-sectional analysis. Longitudinal analyses were not possible because of small numbers: Practically no respondents improved from high levels of impairment (many died, in fact), and not enough became significantly impaired during 3 years of follow-up.

Similar spouse-pair analyses were carried out in an examination of the impact of chronic illness or disability in one spouse on the health and well-being of the other spouse (Kogan, 1987). Table 1.3 highlights the findings. Because of sufficient numbers involving incidence of new conditions or new disability, rigorous longitudinal analyses were possible. These results add valuable new information to the evidence on caregiver burden (Montgomery, 1989).

The psychosocial aspects of the residential environment of the elderly have also been examined in the Yale cohort. One set of analyses concerned themselves with the impact of crime (Berkman,

TABLE 1.2 Impact of Spousal Cognitive Impairment (SPMSQ) on Health and Well-Being of Other Spouse: Cross-Sectional Analyses

Depression
    W impairment increases H depression; adjusted for H age, income, disability, chronic conditions, and W chronic conditions
    No significant effect of H impairment on W depression
High BP or Hypertension
    W impairment increases H BP; adjusted for significant BP correlates; effect stronger on measured BP, weaker on "hypertension" (defined by treatment status); few men treated
    H impairment increases W BP; adjusted for significant BP correlates; effect stronger on "hypertension," weaker on measured BP; most women treated
Self-assessed decline in health ("past year")
    W impairment increases H reports of decline in health
    No significant effect of H impairment on W reports
Alcohol consumption
    Lower consumption if spouse impaired; both sexes
Other effects
    Reliance on spouse for emotional and instrumental support lowered by cognitive impairment; both sexes
    Social and leisure activities outside home: lower if spouse impaired, stronger effect of W impairment on H activities

Note. H = husband; W = wife; BP = blood pressure.

TABLE 1.3 Impact of Spousal Chronic Illness and Disability on Health and Well-Being of Other Spouse

Strategy of data analysis
  For each outcome variable, adjust for all significant correlates (potential confounders)
  For prospective (change) analyses, also adjust for baseline (1982) level of outcome variable
Depression in H
  Cross-sectional: presence of W disability (Katz) and recent bed disability raises H depression
  Prospective: Cancer diagnosis in W (years 82–85) raises H depression
Depression in W
  Cross-sectional: no significant H health variables
  Prospective: heart attack in H (years 82–85) and H cancer history (at baseline) raise W depression
Alcohol consumption by H
  Cross-sectional: W health rated (by W) worse last year raises H consumption (especially if W not the confidant)
  Prospective: none
Alcohol consumption by W
  Cross-sectional: H history of amputation raises W consumption; H health rated (by H) worse last year lowers W consumption
  Prospective: H heart attack (years 82–85) raises W consumption
Sleep problems in H (falling asleep or waking up)
  Cross-sectional: W cataracts, W hospitalized last year, W life-threatening illness (grouped) raise H sleep problems
  Prospective: W disability (Katz), W life-threatening ilness (years 82–85)
Sleep problems in W
  Cross-sectional: H history of arthritis and amputation raise W sleep problems
  Prospective: H heart attack and arthritis (years 82–85) raise W sleep problems
Change (years 82–85) in BP in W
  W disability (Katz) increases H SBP
Change (years 82–85) in BP in W
  H urinary incontinence raises W SBP and DBP; visits from a home health care worker (for H health problem) lowers W SBP

Note. H = husband; W = wife; BP = blood pressure; SBP = systotic blood pressure; DBP = diastolic blood pressure.

1987). Table 1.4 summarizes some of the findings on the impact of being a crime victim. In general, the impact appears to be less than striking; this is reasonably consistent with the general residential literature on the elderly (Kasl & Rosenfield, 1980).

Although the search for an impact of crime victimization was based on an intuitive expectation that this stressor will affect the health and well-being of the elderly, some of our other analyses dealing with the residential environment have been more serendipitous. Table 1.5 illustrates an analysis conducted after we noted some surprising male mortality differences by race and housing stratum (Speechley, Berkman, Singer & Kasl, 1989). There is an excess white male mortality (among the younger old) in the public housing stratum, and it is not

TABLE 1.4 Experience of Being Crime Victim

Question: Have you been a victim of a criminal act (robbery or assault) in the past year (about 6% say "yes")?

Depression
  Men
    Slightly higher depression among victims, not significant in multivariable analysis
  Women
    Significantly higher depression among victims; significant interaction: stronger effect of victimization among social isolates
SBP
  Men and Women
    No effect among normotensives
    Among untreated hypertensives, victims have higher SBP
    Among treated hypertensives, victims have lower SBP
Sleep problems
  Men and women
    No effect
Alcohol consumption
  Men
    No effect
  Women
    Victims more likely to report consumption during "past month"; no difference on amount of consumption; suggests self-selection of those who are drinkers

Note. SBP = systolic blood pressure.

TABLE 1.5 Four-Year Mortality Among New Haven Elderly Men (65–74 Years) by Race and Housing

	Public elderly housing		Community Housing	
	n	% Dying	n	% Dying
White	58	37.9	318	14.8
Black	72	18.1	52	19.2

Note. Higher mortality of white men in public housing particularly striking for those in *better* health. In logistic regression analysis, main effects of housing stratum and race significant as well as housing by race interaction. Adjusted for (a) age, health status and disability, medical care indicators, cognitive impairment; (b) life-style and health habits; (c) sociodemographics and socioeconomic status plus a financial strain index; and (d) network and support variables. Logistic regression coefficient for interaction changes little with progressively elaborated models.

explained by the influence of a large set of potential confounders and explanatory variables. Although the proper interpretation of this finding remains elusive, it does serve to alert us to the need to examine residential parameters in different ways including a global classification of the setting interacting with specific social characteristics acting as vulnerability factors.

Table 1.6 highlights some findings from an earlier study of health effects of relocation (Kasl, Ostfeld, Brody, Snell, & Price, 1980). The negative health impact was evident despite the fact that the move was an improvement in the quality of housing, was not disruptive of social networks, and was associated with higher life satisfaction. This suggests that there are additional parameters of social and residential uprooting that have not yet been spelled out by existing theoretical frameworks and that may point to some fundamental aspects of "attachment to place."

Some of our analyses of the Yale cohort data have involved psychosocial risk factors outside of the normally defined stress domain. One such variable is the respondent's subjective global self-assessment of health (Idler, Kasl, & Lemke, 1990). In analyses that were replicated on elderly men and women, and separately at two sites, New Haven and rural Iowa, it was found that negative self-evaluations of health constituted an independent risk factor for mortality, even after rigorous adjustments for chronic conditions, three measures of disability, sociodemographic characteristics, and health-risk behaviors. In further analyses (Idler & Kasl, 1991), these results were challenged by

TABLE 1.6 Some Consequences of "Involuntary" Relocation Among Poor Urban Elderly After Two Years of Follow-Up

Relocatees (compared with controls)
   More hospitalizations
   Higher incidence of stroke and angina
   More doctor visits (first year only)
   More negative self-evaluation of health
Stronger effects
   If greater anticipatory anxiety about move
   If less of an improvement in the residential environment (dwelling or
     neighborhood)
Results despite following
   Substantial improvement in housing or without greater financial burden
   Little disruption in networks or social interaction
   Higher life satisfaction

including in the logistic regression models additional variables that were potential confounders or potential mediators. Among the former were indexes of medications and history of recent hospitalizations and nursing home stay. Among the latter were several indicators of social support and social networks, the depression scale, and a brief index of optimism (sense of coherence). None of these variables meaningfully altered the regression coefficients reflecting the role of self-assessed health, though some made their own independent prediction of mortality. These results are quite consistent with two previous studies (Kaplan & Camacho, 1983; Mossey & Shapiro, 1982) and suggest that the protective aspects of positive or optimistic self-evaluations of one's health are not due to some broad influences of general well-being and optimism, but are specific to the physical health domain.

We have also begun to explore the role of religion in the health and well-being of the elderly (Idler & Kasl, in press). Table 1.7 shows the results of analyses that reveal the influence of religiousness on course of disability. The latter is measured by a five-level Guttman scale composed of three subscales tapping a range of Activities of Daily Living and physical performance items (for details, see Berkman et al., 1986). Public religiousness reflects attendance at services and congregation members known, whereas private religiousness is based on self-reports of religiousness, and receiving strength and comfort from religion. It can be seen that after adjustments for baseline disability, health status, and other control variables, public religiousness was predictive of a favorable course, whereas private religiousness forecast a declining course. A separate scale of optimism behaved the same way as public religiousness. We are not yet in a position to offer helpful interpretations of these results, though they clearly show the importance of distinguishing the two aspects of religiousness. Public religiousness appears to tap the social dimension of religious involvement and its beneficial effects are specific to religion-related social contacts; Durkheim's (1915/1965) theoretical formulations are most relevant. Private religiousness may indicate a turning inward so that inner peace is the goal, not social role performance and social interaction with others. The turning inward may undermine motivation for recovery or for maintenance of good functioning.

CONCLUSION

A consideration of the psychosocial forces that influence the health of the elderly in modern industrial society cannot escape the presumption of uniqueness of the elderly, which is so much part of our

TABLE 1.7 Role of Religiousness and Optimism in Changes in Disability Among the Elderly

Baseline (1982) variables	1983 Disability		1984 Disability	
	Beta	p	Beta	p
Functional disability at baseline	.400	.000	.397	.000
Age	.027	.000	.041	.000
Female	.057	.427	.190	.003
Physical health index	.063	.000	.077	.000
Exercise	−.166	.000	−.098	.052
Other control variables[a]		n.s.		n.s.
Public religiousness	−.066	.000	−.046	.005
Private religiousness	.064	.045	.098	.001
Optimism	−.050	.000	−.071	.000
Fatalism	.031	.080	.007	.730
Multiple r	.376		.409	
n	1,764		1,662	

[a]Education, income, race, marital status, weight/(height)^2, alcohol consumption, smoking status.

intellectual Zeitgeist. Aside from the presumably universal cultural practice of age grading, there would seem to be at least three other circumstances that reflect and reinforce this presumption: first, the development of academic and scientific disciplines exclusively concerned with the elderly; second, the development of government programs and services targeted on the elderly; and third, the undeniably greater prevalence of adverse conditions among the elderly, particularly those involving economic factors and health status. Perhaps the commonest sequence of these circumstances is the corollary presumption of the greater vulnerability of the elderly.

Similarly, a consideration of the concept of stress and its impact on health taps into the current popular and scientific Zeitgeist of expecting adverse health consequences of exposure to (intuitively selected or theoretically derived) stressors. For example, retirement continues to be viewed as a major stressful life event despite a complete failure to accumulate a mass of credible evidence in favor of such a view (e.g., Goldrick, 1989; Kasl, 1980). Thus, a juxtaposition of the topics of stress and the elderly naturally leads to the presumption that the vulnerability of people in general to stressor effects is greater among the elderly.

It would be wise to adopt the view that presumptions of the uniqueness and vulnerability of the elderly may be an obstacle to a dispassionate examination of the evidence. In fact, we can be comfortable with the general conclusion that the impact of psychosocial factors on health status is not dramatically altered by age. When the evidence suggests that age does act to modify this impact, it is more often seen that the impact is weaker in the elderly than that it is stronger (e.g., Kasl & Berkman, 1981; Seeman, Kaplan, Knudsen, Cohen, & Guralnik, 1987), though comparative evidence across stages of life cycle is extremely fragmentary and often does not allow definitive interpretations. The conclusion that the elderly may not be more vulnerable is perhaps counterintuitive and surprising, because there is much biological evidence suggesting that the elderly are less resilient to stresses, less physiologically adaptable, have slowed homeostatic-regulatory functions, and are less immunologically competent (Finch & Hayflick, 1977; Timiras 1972).

It is possible to offer a perspective that makes the preceding conclusion less surprising, however. This perspective suggests that the health of the elderly person, at any one point, can be seen as a cumulative function of the previous experiences, accumulated over a lifetime.

Any new event comes to represent a diminishing fraction of this total accumulation of events, and the impact thus diminishes proportionally. Of course, this is only a global and incomplete statement of one perspective, and additional assumptions would have to be included and elaborated, such as the process of prior attrition of the more vulnerable; accumulation of past learning facilitating adaptation to the next experience; reduced adaptive demands if societal role expectations become more open-ended; diminishing psychosocial significance of events because of life-cycle changes in aspirations, expectations, and perceptions.

The problem with the preceding perspective is that it can be reasonably invoked after the fact, if the various results support it; however, by itself, it has no compelling theoretical status, and it cannot be an a priori guide to interpreting results. An opposite formulation would be equally convincing if the results favored it—namely, that the elderly are more vulnerable to the impact of various events and experiences because they come to draw on a diminishing or depleted reservoir of adaptive equilibrium or restoring capability (Selye's reservoir of adaptive energy). The subthreshold impact of earlier years cumulates to become the suprathreshold health status change in the elderly.

Although the evidence seems to favor the perspective of a diminishing impact of events and experiences on the health of the elderly, it would also seem that many of us are not comfortable with such a perspective. After all, the elderly seem to live in a state in which mounting social losses, physical debilitation, economic deprivation, and loss of (conventionally defined) useful work activities are occurring with great inevitability, but we do not seem to be able to detect the intuitively expected corresponding impact, such as in clinical depression or physical illnesses (Jarvik, 1976). It is possible, then, that we have an incomplete grasp of the various positive factors in the lives of the elderly—the resources in their social environment and the adaptive strategies available to them—that serve to diminish the impact of the presumptively stressful experiences. Furthermore, we may not have a good understanding of what is specifically stressful to the elderly. That is, if we accept the approximate definition of stress as "demands that tax the adaptive resources," we may well ask if particular events and experiences represent social and personal demands equally for the elderly as for the younger person.

Overall, then, the biological and social sciences dealing with the elderly have accumulated valuable normative data on age-related changes in physiological functioning, health status, and their social conditions. However, these bodies of data cannot be easily juxtaposed to reveal the influence of psychosocial factors in the health of the elderly. We need in particular broader studies of so-called biological aging and secondary aging, which also include psychosocial factors, so that the role of these factors in aging can be assessed more directly.

REFERENCES

Amster, L. E., & Krauss, H. H. (1974). The relationship between life crises and mental deterioration in old age. *International Journal of Aging and Human Development, 5*, 51–55.

Baum, A., Grunberg, N. E., & Singer, J. E. (1982). The use of psychological and neuroendocrinological measurements in the study of stress. *Health Psychology, 1*, 217–236.

Berkman, C. S. (1987). *The impact of crime and safety in the residential environment on the health and well-being of an urban elderly population.* Unpublished doctoral dissertation, Yale University, New Haven, CT.

Berkman, L. F. (1984). Assessing the physical health effects of social networks and social support. *Annual Review of Public Health, 5*, 413–432.

Berkman, L. F., Berkman, C. S., Kasl, S. V., Freeman, D. H., Jr., Leo, L., Ostfeld, A. M., Cornoni-Huntley, J., & Brody, J. A. (1986). Depressive symptoms in relation to physical health and functioning in the elderly. *American Journal of Epidemiology, 124*, 372–388.

Bowling, A. (1987). Mortality after bereavement: A review of the literature on survival periods and factors affecting survival. *Social Science and Medicine, 24*, 117–124.

Chiriboga, D. A. (1989). The measurement of stress exposure in later life. In K. S. Markides & C. L. Cooper (Eds.), *Aging, stress, and health* (pp. 13–41). New York: Wiley & Sons.

Cohen, S. (1986). Contrasting the Hassles Scale and the Perceived Stress Scale: Who's really measuring appraised stress? *American Psychologist, 41*, 716–718.

Cohen, S. (1988). Psychosocial models of the role of social support in the etiology of physical illness. *Health Psychology, 7*, 269–297.

Cohen, S., Kamarck, T., & Mermelstein, R. (1983). A global measure of perceived stress. *Journal of Health and Social Behavior, 24*, 385–396.

Cohen, S., & Syme, S. L. (Eds.). (1985). *Social support and health.* Orlando: Academic Press.

Cook, T. D., & Campbell, D. T. (1979). *Quasi-experimentation: Design & analysis issues for field settings.* Boston: Houghton-Mifflin.

Cornoni-Huntley, J., Brock, D. B., Ostfeld, A. M., Taylor, J. D., & Wallace, R. B. (Eds.). (1986). *Established populations for epidemiologic studies of the elderly* (NIH Publication No. 86-2443). Silver Spring, MD: National Institute on Aging.

Costa, P. T., Jr., & McCrae, R. R. (1989). Personality, stress, and coping: Some lessons from a decade of research. In K. S. Markides, S. Kyriakos, & C. L. Cooper (Eds.), *Aging, stress, and health* (pp. 269–285). New York: Wiley & Sons.

Dohrenwend, B. P., Shrout, P. E., Egri, G., & Mendelsohn, F. S. (1980). Nonspecific psychological distress and other dimensions of psychopathology: Measures for use in the general population. *Archives of General Psychiatry, 37*, 1229–1236.

Durkheim, E. (1965). *The elementary forms of the religious life* (J. W. Swain, Trans.). New York: Free Press. (Original work published 1915)

Finch, C. E., & Hayflick, L. (Eds.). (1977). *Handbook of the biology of aging.* New York: Van Nostrand Reinhold.

Frese, M., & Zapf, D. (1988). Methodological issues in the study of work stress: Objective vs. subjective measurement of work stress and the question of longitudinal studies. In C. L. Cooper & R. Payne (Eds.), *Causes, coping, and consequences of stress at work* (pp. 375–411). New York: Wiley & Sons.

George, L. K. (1980). *Role transitions in later life.* Monterey, CA: Brooks/ Cole.

Goldberg, E. L., & Comstock, G. W. (1980). Epidemiology of life events: Frequency in general populations. *American Journal of Epidemiology, 111*, 736–752.

Goldrick, A. E. (1989). Stress, early retirement, and health. In K. S. Markides & C. L. Cooper (Eds.), *Aging, stress, and health* (pp. 91–118). New York: Wiley & Sons.

Holmes, T. H., & Rahe, R. H. (1967). The social readjustment rating scale. *Journal of Psychosomatic Research, 11*, 213–218.

Houts, P. S., & McDougall, V. (1988). Effects of informing workers of their health risks from exposure to toxic materials. *American Journal of Industrial Medicine, 13*, 271–279.

Idler, E. L., & Kasl, S. V. (1991). Health perceptions and survival: Do global evaluations of health status really predict mortality? *Journal of Gerontology: Social Sciences, 46*, S55–S65.

Idler, E. L., & Kasl, S. V. (in press). Religion, disability, depression and the timing of death. *American Journal of Sociology.*

Idler, E. L., Kasl, S. V., & Lemke, J. H. (1990). Self-evaluated health and mortality among the elderly in New Haven, Connecticut, and Iowa and Washington counties, Iowa, 1982–1986. *American Journal of Epidemiology, 131*, 91–103.

Jarvik, L. F. (1976). Aging and depression: Some unanswered questions. *Journal of Gerontology, 31*, 324–326.

Kanner, A. D., Coyne, J. C., Schaefer, C., & Lazarus, R. S. (1981). Comparisons of two modes of stress measurement: Daily hassles and uplifts versus major life events. *Journal of Behavioral Medicine, 4*, 1–39.

Kaplan, G. A., & Camacho, T. (1983). Perceived health and mortality: A nine-year follow-up of the Human Population Laboratory cohort. *American Journal of Epidemiology, 117*, 292–304.

Kasl, S. V. (1980). The impact of retirement. In C. L. Cooper & R. Payne (Eds.), *Current concerns in occupational stress* (pp. 137–186). New York: Wiley & Sons.

Kasl, S. V. (1983). Pursuing the link between stressful life experiences and disease: A time for re-appraisal. In C. L. Cooper (Ed.), *Stress research* (pp. 79–102). New York: Wiley & Sons.

Kasl, S. V. (1984a). Stress and health. *Annual Review of Public Health, 5*, 319–341.

Kasl, S. V. (1984b). When to welcome a new measure. *American Journal of Public Health, 74*, 106–108.

Kasl, S. V. (1985). Environmental exposure and disease: An epidemiological perspective on some methodological issues in health psychology and behavioral medicine. In A. Baum & J. E. Singer (Eds.), *Advances in environmental psychology* (Vol. 5): *Methods and environmental psychology* (pp. 119–146). Hillsdale, NJ: Erlbaum.

Kasl, S. V. (1989). An epidemiological perspective on the role of control in health. In S. L. Sauter, J. J. Hurrell, Jr., & C. L. Cooper (Eds.), *Job control and worker health* (pp. 161–189). New York: Wiley & Sons.

Kasl, S. V., & Berkman, L. F. (1981). Some psychosocial influences on the health status of the elderly. In J. L. McGaugh & S. V. Kiesler (Eds.), *Aging: Biology and behavior* (pp. 345–385). New York: Academic Press.

Kasl, S. V., Ostfeld, A. M., Berkman, L. F., & Jacobs, S. C. (1987). Stress and alcohol consumption: The role of selected social and environmental factors. In E. Gottheil, K. A. Druley, S. Pashko, & S. P. Weinstein (Eds.), *Stress and addiction* (pp. 40–60). New York, Brunner/Mazel.

Kasl, S. V., Ostfeld, A. M., Brody, G. M., Snell, L., & Price, C. A. (1980). Effects of "involuntary" relocation on the health and behavior of the elderly. In S. G. Haynes & M. Feinleib (Eds.), *Second conference on the epidemiology of aging: Proceedings of the second conference* (NIH Publication No. 80-969) (pp. 211–232). Bethesda, MD: U.S. Department of Health and Human Services.

Kasl, S. V., & Rosenfield, S. (1980). The residential environment and its impact on the mental health of the aged. In J. E. Birren & R. B. Sloane (Eds.), *Handbook of mental health and aging* (pp. 468–498). Englewood Cliffs, NJ: Prentice Hall.

Kogan, M. D. (1987). *The impact on the health status of the spouse due to chronic illness and disability in the partner.* Unpublished doctoral dissertation, Yale University, New Haven, CT.

Markides, K. S., & Cooper, C. L. (Eds.). (1989). *Aging, stress, and health.* New York: Wiley & Sons.

Masuda, M., & Holmes, T. H. (1978). Life events: Perceptions and frequencies. *Psychosomatic Medicine, 40,* 236–269.

McGrath, J. E. (1970). A conceptual formulation for research on stress. In J. E. McGrath (Ed.), *Social and psychological factors in stress* (pp. 10–21). New York: Holt, Rinehart and Winston.

Mendes de Leon, C. F., Kasl, S. V., & Jacobs, S. (1991). Widowhood and mortality risk in a community sample of the elderly: A prospective study. Manuscript submitted for publication.

Montgomery, R. J. (1989). Investigating caregiver burden. In K. S. Markides & C. L. Cooper (Eds.), *Aging, stress, and health* (pp. 201–218). New York: Wiley & Sons.

Moritz, D. J. (1987). *The health impact of living with cognitively impaired elderly spouse.* Unpublished doctoral dissertation, Yale University, New Haven, CT.

Moritz, D. J., Kasl, S. V., & Berkman, L. F. (1989). The health impact of living with a cognitively impaired spouse: Depressive symptoms and social functioning. *Journal of Gerontology: Social Sciences, 44,* 517–527.

Mossey, J. M., & Shapiro, E. (1982). Self-rated health: A predictor of mortality among the elderly. *American Journal of Public Health, 72,* 800–808.

Murrell, S. A., & Himmelfarb, S. (1989). Effects of attachment bereavement and pre-event conditions on subsequent depressive symptoms in older adults. *Psychology and Aging, 4,* 166–172.

Murrell, S. A., Norris, F. H., & Hutchins, G. L. (1984). Distribution and desirability of life events in older adults: Population and policy implications. *Journal of Community Psychology, 12,* 301–311.

Pearlin, L. I., Lieberman, M. A., Menaghan, E. G., & Mullan, J. T. (1982). The stress process. *Journal of Health and Social Behavior, 22,* 337–356.

Pfeiffer, E. (1975). A short portable mental status questionnaire for the assessment of organic brain deficit in elderly patients. *Journal of the American Geriatrics Society, 22,* 433–441.

Phifer, J. F., Kaniasty, K. Z., & Norris, F. H. (1988). The impact of natural disaster on the health of older adults: A multiwave prospective study. *Journal of Health and Social Behavior, 29,* 65–78.

Radloff, L. S. (1977). The CES-D scale: A self-report depression scale for research in the general population. *Journal of Applied Psychological Measurement, 1,* 385–401.

Rodin, J. (1986). Health, control and aging. In M. M. Baltes & P. B. Baltes

(Eds.), *The psychology of control and aging* (pp. 139–165). Hillsdale, NJ: Erlbaum.

Rodin, J., Timko, C., & Harris, S. (1985). The construct of control: Biological and psychosocial correlates. *Annual Review of Gerontology and Geriatrics, 5,* 3–55.

Sarason, I. G., & Sarason, B. R. (Eds.). (1985). *Social support: Theory, research, and applications.* Boston: Martinus Nijhoff.

Sauter, S. L., Hurrell, J. J., Jr., & Cooper, C. L. (Eds.). (1989). *Job control and worker health.* New York: Wiley & Sons.

Seeman, T. E., Kaplan, G. A., Knudsen, L., Cohen, R., & Guralnik, J. (1987). Social network ties and mortality among the elderly in the Alameda County Study. *American Journal of Epidemiology, 126,* 714–723.

Selye, H. (1983). The stress concept: Past, present, and future. In C. L. Cooper (Ed.), *Stress research* (pp. 1–20). New York: Wiley & Sons.

Shumaker, S. A., & Czajkowski, S. M. (Eds.). (in press). *Social support and cardiovascular disease.* New York: Plenum.

Speechley, M., Berkman, L. F., Singer, B. H., & Kasl, S. V. *Housing and race effects in mortality among New Haven elderly, 1982–1986.* Unpublished manuscript, Yale University School of Medicine, Department of Epidemiology and Public Health, New Haven.

Speers, M. A., Kasl, S. V., Freeman, D. H., Jr., & Ostfeld, A. M. (1986). Blood pressure concordance between spouses. *American Journal of Epidemiology, 123,* 818–829.

Timiras, P. (1972). *Developmental physiology and aging.* New York: MacMillan.

Tobin, S. S., & Lieberman, M. A. (1976). *Last home for the aged.* San Francisco: Jossey-Bass.

Watson, D., & Pennebaker, J. W. (1989). Health complaints, stress, and distress: Exploring the central role of negative affectivity. *Psychological Review, 96,* 234–254.

2

Paradise Lost: Stress in the Modern Age

David A. Chiriboga

The title of this chapter refers to a condition facing many researchers who seek to understand better how stress affects our lives: a condition of having lost paradise. Paradise in this case, however, does not refer to some lost Eden but to a seemingly ideal world in which simple but powerful measures existed of simple but powerful constructs. These constructs dealt with the nature and meaning of stress, a topic around which successive approaches to definition and measurement seemed eminently successful, for a time. Understanding these ever-changing approaches holds particular importance to gerontology, a field that deals with populations often exposed to stressful life circumstances.

WORLD OF STRESS: THEN AND NOW

During the years since the early 1940s, stress research has undergone several major evolutions in what amount to successive paradigm shifts. In fact, there seem to have been three generations of stress research during the past 20 to 25 years. The three generations could be categorized as those of catastrophe research, life-event research, and research on the stressors of everyday life. We may even be on the verge of developing a fourth, and more integrative, model that incorporates properties of those that have preceded it.

The following sections review the way we were and the way we seem to be today, in the world of stress and coping, and conclude with a few comments about where we seem to be heading. From the perspective of gerontology, one point of interest is that for many years gerontologists essentially followed the mainstream of stress research, borrowing concepts and principles as needed. Today, however, gerontologists have emerged as one of the leading, and most active, forces in stress research.

Another point to remember is that each approach to be reviewed is still actively pursued, albeit in somewhat modified form. The reason is that each approach held, and continues to hold, considerable promise. One conclusion of this chapter, in fact, is that the most productive approach represents an integration of all those that have preceded.

CATASTROPHE RESEARCH

The earliest sustained efforts at investigating stress, through catastrophe research, used an approach typified by the study of persons who had experienced extremely disruptive life circumstances. Catastrophe research considers primary effects of one major stressor on an individual and does not only refer to sequelae of extreme stress, such as holocaust survivor research. The intellectual origins of this approach could be said to lie in early psychoanalytic theory, in which a principle concern was with reactions to extreme duress (e.g., Breuer & Freud, 1955). Lindemann's (1944) research on the impact of the Coconut Grove disaster, and Grinker and Spiegel's (1963) classic study of American soldiers in World War II serve as early and pace-setting examples of this genre of stress research. Even Selye (1956), the self-avowed "father" of stress research, could be said to follow this research model, because his research design generally included rather devastatingly (to his animal subjects) invasive physical trauma. Research methods rely heavily on categorization of subjects' response to a single event. Instruments tend toward open-ended questions; in more recent research, coping scales have been used.

Stress as a Given

In the typical study following the catastrophe model, it is accepted as a given that the subjects are, or were, subjected to extremely distressing life circumstances. The underlying question concerns how individuals fare, given their exposure to high levels of stress.

Relocation Stress: Early Focus of Research in Aging

An example taken from gerontological studies concerns the nature and meaning of relocation. As early as the 1920s, concerns were being raised about the impact of involuntary relocation on older persons (e.g., Pollack, 1925). Later, Aldrich and Mendkoff (1963) showed an increase in mortality 1 year following institutionalization, whereas Lieberman, Prock and Tobin (1968) examined the more psychological reactions to institutionalization. These early studies pointed to the often extreme and pervasive debilitation of older relocatees.

As has been the case with much catastrophe research, the assumption usually was made that environmental change is a major stressor to older persons. Evidence gradually accumulated concerning the importance of both the quality and quantity of information people were given about their new home, how positively or negatively they perceived the relocation, and how much control they felt they had over the situation. Even for people involved in the same relocation, as in the specific case of a mass dispersal of individuals from one institution to another, marked differences were found in how individuals viewed and reacted to the situation (Chiriboga, 1972). In early as well as more recent studies (e.g., Pruchno & Resch, 1989; Tobin & Lieberman, 1976), however, the focus of research has been on mediating factors and outcomes rather than on how to assess the actual stress context. That is, the degree of stressfulness of the relocation is often taken for granted rather than being cast as a variable worthy of study in its own right.

Posttraumatic Stress Disorder

Given its focus on the aftermath and not the event, it is not surprising that one contribution of catastrophe research has been an increased understanding of victims. The clinical study of people who have suffered extreme stress has become a major interest. More than 20 years ago the Center for the Study of Neurosis was developed by Horowitz (1986). A more recent example is the San Diego Center for Prisoner of War Research (Hunter, 1988). One result of such attention has been the identification of a specific grouping of symptoms as being related to exposure to extreme stress conditions, described in the third edition of the *Diagnostic Statistical Manual of Mental Disorders* (American Psychiatric Association, 1980).

Clinicians have not only described a series of reactions to extreme stress that may unfold but have advanced approaches to therapeutic intervention. The interventions described are generally focused on facilitating the progression of what is viewed as the unfolding of a stress-response syndrome (e.g., Golan, 1978; Horowitz, 1986; Noshpitz & Coddington, 1990). The work of Kubler-Ross (1969), depicting stages of resolving the reality of impending death, represents an approach to the study of coping that focuses on the process of working through problems associated with a devastating stressor.

Whether viewed as a stress response or as a general description of how people deal with devastating conditions, one rather remarkable fact is the similarity in how clinical researchers have described behavior following major stress. As portrayed by Kubler-Ross (1969), Tyhurst (1957), Horowitz (1986), and many others, the stages of the stress response, in general, can be characterized as consisting of (a) emotional numbing, (b) outcry and anger, (c) denial, (d) intrusive thoughts, (e) working through, and (f) resolution and acceptance. These stages would seem applicable to persons of any age.

Enhanced Risk of the Elderly

From the early work of Friedsam (1960) to the present (Phifer, 1990), researchers have emphasized the special vulnerabilities of the elderly to various catastrophic conditions. Although much of the early work was concerned primarily with the impact of environmental change of one kind or another, conditions such as bereavement, exposure to natural disasters, onset of various cancer, and other health problems have also been addressed. A few gerontologists are now also looking at the more positive side—what makes for "good" or "hardy" copers in later life (e.g., Aldwin & Revenson, 1987; Fiske & Chiriboga, 1990; Kahana, Harel, & Kahana, 1988).

Coping: Another Way of Viewing the Stress-Response Syndrome

Although much of the catastrophe-oriented research has focused on stress responses, there is growing interest on a closely related topic: the ways in which people cope with highly distressful conditions. An extensive literature, in fact, has developed around how people cope with a multitude of life stressors, some major and some not so major. One continuing problem in this literature has been disagreement about whether coping refers to behavior directed toward alleviation of a specific stressful situation, to general personality traits, to defense mechanisms, or to some combination of all of these. At the most general level, the word "coping" can refer to any activity aimed at reducing distress, or to only those behaviors and qualities associated with the actual alleviation of distress (Kahana et al., 1988; Lazarus & Folkman, 1984; Pearlin, Menaghan, Lieberman & Mullan, 1981).

Of particular interest is that researchers working within the broad domain of catastrophe research, both currently and in the past, have frequently come up with what appear to be basic predispositions toward coping activities. For example, Cohen and Lazarus (1973) identified two basic groups—copers and avoiders—whereas Janis (1958) described people who in response to a surgical intervention reacted with either denial or information seeking. More recently, Miller (1980b) has described monitors and blunters as two predisposing types that may characterize individuals of any age.

Within the field of gerontology, there has long been an interest in the topic of coping styles. The earliest and most sustained work has been conducted by Gutmann (1964) with middle-aged and older adults. Studying such diverse groups as the nomadic Druze of the Middle East; the Navajo of Arizona; and white, middle-class residents of Kansas City, Gutmann found evidence for the existence of at least three distinct styles of dealing with the world: an active mastery style in which the individual takes an active and assertive stance, a passive mastery style in which individuals are characteristically accommodating to demands imposed on them, and a magical mastery style in which individuals attempt to cope with situations through denial and unusual redefinitions of the situation. Based on interpretations of classic projection tests, his results indicated that middle-aged men most often can be characterized as manifesting an active mastery style, whereas passive mastery becomes more typical in the later years. Conversely, women from all cultures seemed to move from a more passive style of mastery to one emphasizing active mastery.

Although Gutmann's work (1964, 1985) has been criticized for its reliance on clinical interpretations, some corroborating evidence has been found in empirical studies. Lowenthal, Thurnher, and Chiriboga (1975), for example, report that middle-aged men demonstrated a more masterful and instrumental sense of self, on the basis of an adjective checklist, whereas those approaching the retirement years were seemingly more attuned to accommodation and valuation of the needs of others. Similarly, in studying the coping strategies of older persons in long-term care facilities, Quayhagen and Chiriboga (1976) found that passive styles of coping predominated. The suggestion, drawn from all these studies, that older adults employ more passive styles of coping is especially provocative.

Coping with Divorce: Example of Catastrophe Research

Although divorce is often viewed as a crisis or transition of young adulthood, it is experienced by increasing numbers of middle-aged and older adults (Chiriboga, Catron, & Associates, 1991). The study of divorce also includes at least one of the hallmarks of traditional catastrophe research: Subjects share the experience of what most people would agree is a devastating situation. In one investigation conducted in the San Francisco Bay Area, men and women were interviewed within 8 months of marital separation and then again approximately 3.5 years later. The random sample, drawn from county clerk records, included individuals ranging in age from 20 to mid-70s and therefore provided a life-span, if not gerontological, perspective on divorce.

Moreover, the disparity between the more common factor-derived coping studies and the global portrayal of coping styles evident in the work of Gutmann (1964, 1985) and others forced the research team to resort to a rather uncommon analytical strategy. The analytical strategy was to develop an empirical typology of coping styles. Both gerontologists and stress researchers in general have tended to follow a similar approach to studying coping: Data from a structured instrument are subjected to some factor extraction technique that is coupled to an orthogonal rotation, and the resulting factors are used as indexes of coping. This approach seemed, to the research team at least, to possess a critical flaw: It ignores the fact that individuals possess all the coping strategies, at one level or another, and that the overall profile on these strategies may be critical to the efficacy of the strategies.

Until recently the statistical procedure, cluster analysis, associated with empirical typologies has been missing from common statistical packages. Now available in both SPSS and SAS, cluster analysis allowed us to identify specific styles of coping that are reflected in particular combinations of individual coping strategies. The first step was to run a factor analysis, with oblique rotation, of the 68-item Lazarus and Folkman (1984) Ways of Coping Scale. This analysis yielded eight factors that were considered as "building blocks" for coping (Chiriboga et al., 1991).

The eight factors fell nicely within a schema posed by Pearlin and Schooler (1978), according to whom coping behaviors are divided into those directed at altering the problem situation, those that seek to redefine or indirectly alter the situation, and those whose goal is managing the stress response. The factors that represented situation altering behaviors included help seeking and active mastery. The two factors that represented situation redefining and other indirect behaviors were growth and wish-fulfilling fantasy.

The remaining four factors dealt with management of emotions, and included the only two for which significant age effects were found. One factor suggested the use of cognitive strategies and was labeled cognitive control. The others dealt in one fashion or another with emotional-focused behaviors. Emotive action generally dealt with both accepting and releasing one's feelings; younger men and women were more likely to use this strategy than those aged 40 and older. Self-blame involved a blaming or self-critical attitude. Fatalism ("Went along with fate; sometimes you just have bad luck," or "Accepted it, since nothing could be done") was of particular interest because it bears resemblance to Gutmann's (1964) passive mastery style. Divorcing men in their 40s were the lowest on this strategy, whereas women in the 40s were the most fatalistic.

Profiles of Coping

To determine whether they shared similar profiles or "styles" of coping, the divorce study subjects were grouped according to a cluster analysis program that assigns subjects according to common profiles of scores and also makes few distributional assumptions (Tryon & Bailey, 1970).

Seven coping styles were identified (Chiriboga et al., 1991). The first type we called *noncopers*. The 21 noncopers scored the lowest, or equal to the lowest, on seven of the coping strategies. They were intermediate only on self-blame; that is, they were more likely to blame themselves than were some other groups.

Two coping styles were significantly higher than the rest on the situation-altering factors of help seeking and active mastery, but differed from each other on most of the remaining strategies. One style, labeled *action copers*, included persons ($n = 37$) high on help seeking and active mastery, but generally low on the situation redefining and stress-management coping strategies. The second action-oriented style, labeled *supercopers*, consisted of persons ($n = 41$) who not only were high on help seeking and active mastery, but on most of the other factors as well. Supercopers were intermediate only on self-blame and fantasy, two strategies that the literature suggests as being associated with greater symptomatology.

The 19 *mystics* scored highest in the perception of stress as a growth possibility. They were high on fatalism and emotive action, but low to intermediate on all other strategies. The 32 *stoics* shared with the mystics the quality of being high in fatalism and emotive action. Although the mystics were also highly optimistic about the growth-promoting possibilities in their situation, the stoics were the highest on a stress-management strategy: cognitive control. That is, they were the most likely of all types to use selective ignoring as a coping strategy—a strategy that Pearlin and Schooler (1978) found to be the least effective mediator of stress.

The *balanced* style consisted of 29 persons who generally fell in the intermediate region on all strategies. In essence they were "middle of the roaders" as far as coping is concerned. Finally, the 36 *imaginative copers* scored in the intermediate range on the situation-altering and situation-redefining strategies but were extremely high on self-blame and wish-fulfilling fantasy.

This examination of the coping styles used by divorced men and women indicates considerable diversity in how people sought to handle stressful situations. The action copers, for example, were a relatively pure situation-altering group. In this, they stood in contrast to the supercopers, who were high not only in situation-altering behaviors but on nearly everything else as well.

The noncopers, again in contrast, tended not to use any of the coping strategies included in the 68-item Ways of Coping Scale. Then there were the imaginative copers, highest on strategies, self-blame, and fantasy that analyses with other samples (Chiriboga & Bailey, 1989) have indicated as maladaptive. The mystics and stoics resembled each other closely on all strategies except that mystics were higher on the growth approach to redefining situations, whereas stoics were high in cognitive control, an emotion-focused strategy. The balanced stood out only as people who in fact did not stand out, but instead scored in the more or less average range for each strategy.

Relevance of Coping Style

Identifying coping style is just the first step in analyses of this sort. The next step is to determine whether the styles tell us anything meaningful about the well-being of people. We did this by examining differences in basic socioeconomic and divorce-related characteristics such as age, gender, socioeconomic status, length of marriage, number of children, reported ease of separation, and a summary score for how many life events were reported. Significant differences were found only for age (Chiriboga et al., 1991). The noncopers, people who scored low on all eight strategies, were the oldest, with an average age of approximately 40 years. The active copers were next oldest—they averaged 36 years—and the remaining groups were not significantly different.

How persons within each coping style differed in adaptive status at follow-up was more crucial to our understanding. Adaptive status was assessed by a count of symptoms from the California Symptoms Checklist (Lowenthal et al., 1975), how happy they reported themselves to be, and positive and negative emotions experienced in the week preceding the interview (Bradburn & Caplovitz, 1965). For 5 of these 14 measures of adaptation, the following significant differences were found (Chiriboga et al., 1991):

1. The least lonely were the active copers and the supercopers, with the most lonely being the imaginative copers.
2. Active copers and the balanced were the least likely to report feeling they could not get going, whereas the imaginative escapers were the most likely.
3. The least depressed were the active copers, supercopers, and the Mystics, whereas those reporting feeling most depressed were the imaginative escapers.
4. The noncopers, active copers, and balanced were the least likely to feel uneasy; the most likely to feel this way were the imaginative escapers.
5. The active copers had the fewest psychological symptoms, whereas the imaginative escapers and stoics reported the most.

There was also a tendency for the active copers, supercopers, and Mystics to be the happiest at follow-up, and for the noncopers and imaginative escapers to be the least happy.

Overall, these results suggest that the study of coping styles, as distinguished from studying separate and distinct coping strategies, may add to our understanding of the stress process and how it evolves. The analytical approach, cluster analysis, is also suggested as worthy of consideration by those interested in grouping subjects according to some limited range of characteristics. Although rarely encountered in American research, cluster analysis is widely used in studies conducted in Great Britain.

Advantages of Catastrophe Research

One of the clearest advantages of the more catastrophe-oriented studies of stress is that, regardless of how the situation is perceived by individuals, one may hypothesize that the individuals are indeed facing a potentially distressing context. Much of what we know about coping strategies and styles has been gathered in studies using a catastrophe framework, assuming the event experienced was very stressful. This assumption may be invalid, however, especially when dealing with older adults. The latter have been found to generally experience fewer life events than younger adults (Fiske & Chiriboga, 1990; Horowitz & Wilner, 1980), although the ones they do experience may be of greater severity. Traditional assumptions about the magnitude of stress perceived in particular life styles may be erroneous in older populations. Indeed, boredom, the absence of events, was a frequent complaint in at least one study of older, working-class adults (Fiske & Chiriboga, 1990). Long periods of routine, interrupted by occasional crises involving social loss or physical health, characterized their lives.

Disadvantages of Catastrophe Research

As may have become clear to the reader, the scope of catastrophe research is extremely broad. For example, this genre covers not only the rather acute crisis precipitated by exposure to a natural disaster like a tornado or perhaps Chernobyl or Three Mile Island, but also exposure to situations such as internment in a concentration camp or the slowly unfolding death of oneself or a loved one. This breadth and diversity makes it difficult to pinpoint disadvantages (as well as advantages) of the approach, but several general problems exist.

Heterogeneity of Response

It has been noted several times earlier that studies subsumed under this model often assume that the stressful experience is essentially equivalent across subjects. In other words, all individuals who have been through the same crisis situation, whether it be a flood, bereavement, or relocation, are faced with a similar context and perceive the situation in the same way.

Conversely, stress researchers have found marked variations in how people respond to what on the surface would seem to be the same condition. As an example, the author recalls a graduate student who pointed out an apparent error in a life-events protocol: a middle-aged woman had checked off the death of her spouse as a positive event. On investigation, it turned out that she was a devout Catholic whose spouse had suffered from a prolonged and very painful rectal cancer for more than 2 years. The husband's death was seen as a relief from his sufferings: He was going to a better place, where sometime in the future she would join him.

The point is what appears to be a similar situation, whether it be exposure to a fire fight in Operation Desert Storm, involuntary relocation of a dependent senior, or learning one has incurable cancer, may be perceived in many different ways by different people. To assume that they all perceive the situation in the same way can lead to misinterpretations of how and where they end up.

Postevent Designs

The focus of catastrophe research is generally on what happens to people after the experience of some devastating experience, rather than before. This is due, in large part, to the difficulty in identifying people who will subsequently experience a major stressor. The life-span study of divorce, described earlier, would have required a sample of more than 4,000 if the intent were to study couples before as well as after separation. For similar reasons, studies of bereavement rarely if ever begin before the death of the spouse or child. Studies of how people react to the prospect of their own death, as another example, rarely start with a larger group of persons in apparent good health, some of whom will die in the future. Most catastrophe designs are therefore generally post hoc (Baum, 1987), although stressors such as relocations or hurricanes may on occasion provide sufficient lead time to permit sampling before the event.

Sampling Problems with Collection of Information

Several criticisms have been raised regarding sampling. For example, Baum (1987) notes the difficulty in assessing people who have just experienced a devastating event, both in terms of identifying such people and in getting them to cooperate. Moreover, it is frequently difficult to identify any kind of a reasonable control or comparison group—a problem that accentuates the frequent lack of baseline or prestress data.

Rarity of Stress Condition

Catastrophe research generally focuses on relatively rare conditions that are difficult to sample. Moreover, given both the presumed severity, and the rarity, of the conditions, there is a question concerning how much we learn about the stressors most people face, from the study of unusual conditions.

New Generation of Catastrophe Researchers

The late 1980s and early 1990s have witnessed the emergence of a new cohort of clinicians and researchers who are following catastrophe models of research, although in somewhat modified fashion. This newer generation tends to focus on extreme stressors and their consequences for victims. One consistent topic has been the plight of persons who have suffered from physical and psychological trauma associated with problems such as rape, breast cancer, and even the long-term sequelae of internment in Nazi concentration camps or of the prisoner of war experience. Studies of stress experiences among nursing home residents might be a comparable example.

This new cohort of people who might be classified as catastrophe researchers include people like Wortman and Silver (1987), Dunkel-Schetter (1984), Hobfoll (1988), Taylor and Dakof (1988), and Miller (in press). Miller, for example, is looking at people she calls monitors and blunters, who have characteristic ways of dealing with stressful situations. Taylor and Dakof (1988) and Singer (1988) are studying, among other topic areas, the ways in which people deal with breast cancer. Hobfoll (1988) has dealt extensively with the impact of war on civilian populations.

The continuing interest in catastrophe research is also evident among gerontologists. Kahana et al. (1988), for example, have examined the continuing significance of the Holocaust for people now entering the later stages of life. The burgeoning research on the plight of caregivers to dependent older persons (e.g., Brody, 1989; Deimling, Bass, Townsend, & Noelker, 1989) also represents a variation of the catastrophe model, with the bulk of the research focusing on how people deal with the burden of caring.

Overall, then, we can see that there are distinct advantages as well as disadvantages to the catastrophe model of stress research. Probably the most limiting factor of the approach, in at least its "pure" form, is that the design does not seem relevant to the study of the problems of ordinary men and women. Problems encountered in applying the methodology to the study of anything but essentially infrequent and uniquely distressing situations led to another research strategy: the study of life events.

LIFE-EVENTS RESEARCH

The so-called life events approach to stress research got its start in the mid-1960s. The first instruments were relatively simple and brief inventories of situations that persons might encounter. Antonovsky et al. (1965) generated among the first of this type for a general audience, while Lowenthal, Berkman, and Associates (1967) produced a brief inventory for use with older adults. In both cases, respondents simply checked those items that they had experienced, and the researchers simply tallied the number of events.

Although the apparent reduction in stressful experiences in older samples may to some extent be an artifact of instrument insensitivity, those interested in how older adults deal with stressful experiences should consider the lower rate of life events when selecting samples. Studying stress in samples unlikely to experience stress could lead to some frustration. In a ground-breaking panel study of stress among middle-class, middle-aged men and women, for example, Lazarus and colleagues (Richard Lazarus, personal communication, October 5, 1990) found that subjects were generally not undergoing stressors of any major consequence. This was not a serious problem for the researchers, because the focus of that study was on day-to-day hassles and uplifts. It may have influenced the results, however. For example, one conclusion reached in the study was that day-to-day hassles exert more of an impact on well-being than do life events (DeLongis, Coyne, Dakof, Folkman, & Lazarus, 1982; Lazarus & Folkman, 1984). This would not be surprising in a population that in fact rarely experienced life events.

Schedule of Recent Life Events (SRE)

Life-events research received its major impetus from the publication of reports based on what seemed at the time to be an ideal instrument: the well-known Schedule of Recent Events (Holmes & Rahe, 1967), which was widely used with all age groups. For a period of approximately 10 to 15 years after its introduction, the SRE was the instrument of choice for stress research. A 42-item inventory of life events, the SRE included a sophisticated weighting system based on the assumption that each life event imposed on people a more or less standard demand for readjustment. The SRE was also readily comprehensible to both researchers and subjects, and quick to administer.

Other Event Inventories

Perhaps the most widely accepted alternate to the SRE is the PERI Life Events Scale. The Psychiatric Epidemiology Research Interview (PERI) is one of the more comprehensive or omnibus event inventories, in that it includes 102 items and is intended to have life-span applicability. In fact, although the PERI scale was not designed specifically for an older population, a review of the scale suggests that only three items were probably impossible for an older person to experience: "entered the armed services," "became pregnant," and "abortion."

SRE-Type Instruments for Older Populations

One advantage of instruments based on the SRE approach is that they are fairly readily adapted for use with specialized populations, such as surgical patients, graduate students, or older persons. The adaptability of the SRE in fact has led to several revisions designed for use with older populations. In one of the first such revisions, Amster and Krauss (1974) removed several items and added several including reaching the age of 65. Because they provided little rationale for the new items, their instrument has received little or no attention. Other revisions have fared somewhat better. Mensh (1983), for example, has developed a 27-item modification with promise, as have Kahana, Kahana, and Young (1987) (see also Aldwin & Revenson, 1987; Kiyak, Liang & Kahana, 1976).

Other Event Inventories for Older Populations

PERI Life Events Scale

This scale is used in its full version by some gerontologists, whereas others have shortened the instrument. Cohen, Teresi, and Holmes (1985), for example, reduced the scale to 15 items. Modifications to the scale are not always as drastic. In an effort to create a more age-relevant instrument, Krause (1986a, 1986b) reduced the PERI scale but added items from other scales. The resulting 77-item inventory groups events into categories involving children, spouse, other relatives, friends, neighborhood, finances, crime, and miscellaneous. Using simple tallies of reported life events, as opposed to the standard weights developed by Dohrenwend, Krasnoff, Askenasy, & Dohrenwend (1978), Krause has found his modification to have good construct and predictive validity.

Louisville Older Persons Events Scale (LOPES)

LOPES was developed by Murrell, Norris, and Hutchins (1984), and Murrell, Norris, and Grote (1987) as a broad-spectrum life-events inventory for older persons. With 54 items selected on the basis of extensive pretesting with older populations (e.g., Murrell et al., 1984), LOPES elicits information on life events experienced during a shorter period, 6 months, than is usually the case with event inventories. One consequence of this shorter time-span may be greater reliability of recall. The instrument also requests information on more characteristics of each event than is usual or perhaps even necessary for most research needs: desirability, degree of continued preoccupation, date, and novelty.

Lewinsohn Event Inventories

Lewinsohn and his colleagues have developed several stress inventories that are relevant to studies of older populations. The Pleasant Events Schedule (PES) was developed on the basis of reports by subjects primarily of college age but included older individuals as well (Lewinsohn & MacPhillamy, 1974). Teri and Lewinsohn (1982) have revised this instrument by considering impact and frequency of occurrence among subjects ranging in age from 50 to 97 years. The shorter version, labeled the PES-Elderly, contains 114 items, but retains the original tally of frequency and ratings on how enjoyable each event was. Sample items include "being in the country, laughing, kissing, taking a nap, being with my grandchildren, and traveling."

The Unpleasant Events Schedule (UES) is designed to assess the frequency and unpleasantness of 320 events reported in extensive pilot testing to be generally aversive in nature (Lewinsohn, Mermelstein, Alexander & MacPhillamy, 1985; Lewinsohn & Talkington, 1979). The instrument has been used extensively in studies of depression, for which it has demonstrated worth as a predictor (e.g., Lewinsohn et al., 1985). As was the case in the development of the PES, however, the UES instrument development phase drew largely on undergraduate populations, and the bulk of the items are not particularly relevant to middle-aged and older adults. The UES was subsequently reduced in length to 131 items, using the same procedures followed in shortening the PES. Sample items include "being alone, receiving junk mail, death of an acquaintance, shopping for daily necessities, owing money, having my pet sicken and die" (Teri & Lewinsohn, 1982, p. 445).

Despite efforts to expand the range of items, a major limitation of most of these measuring tools is the adequacy of their content, given the diversity of life events that may be encountered during later life and the general lack of systematic attempts to identify suitable content.

Anticipated Stress

As noted by Kemeny, Cohen, Zegans, and Conant (1989), one interesting modification of the typical life-events approach is to ask respondents to check off events that are anticipated to happen within a specific interval as well as rate the degree of distress or worry they were experiencing as a result of expecting the event to occur. Anticipated life stress was found to be significantly associated with reduced numbers of T cells of the immune system.

Stress Exposure and Process of Divorce

The life-event genre of stress research can be illustrated with results from the previously mentioned panel study of divorce. This study in fact used a "catastrophe" strategy to identify subjects but did not make the assumption of equal experience. Included among the instruments was a rather lengthy life-event instrument, developed in collaboration with Mardi Horowitz and Richard Rahe, both research psychiatrists. One goal of the divorce study was to identify stressors that were unique to the transition of divorce as compared with stressors arising as a result of other life circumstances. Another goal was to consider in which ways our older respondents experienced fewer or greater stressors when compared with younger respondents.

We first looked at age and gender differences on 22 stress measures. These measures were derived from a 138-item life events questionnaire (Chiriboga, 1977; Chiriboga & Dean, 1978) that represented an expansion of the Holmes and Rahe (1967) Schedule of Recent Events. The 22 measures consisted of positive and negative scores on 11 different dimensions of stress: dating and marital, family, work, legal, leisure, habits, internal events (e.g., not achieving an important goal), nonfamily relationships, personal (e.g., discrimination, changes in religious beliefs), financial, home and school. Summary scores for positive and negative stress were also computed, as was a ratio of positive to negative stress.

Negative Life Events

There were no age differences, across all 11 dimensions, in experiences with negative stressors. This similarity is surprising, because most studies that include young adult and middle-aged and older adults have found significant declines in stress exposure after young adulthood (e.g., Chiriboga, 1984; Horowitz & Wilner, 1980; Masuda & Holmes, 1978). One possibility is that marital separation increases the levels of stress reported by middle-aged respondents over and above the increase found in young adults, to the point that the usual exposure gap is closed.

Not only were the younger and older respondents the same, but all scored highest in the same two negative dimensions: dating and marital, and internal (Chiriboga et al., 1991). Because these two dimensions contain items applicable to the divorce process, this concentration of events was not entirely unexpected. It may simply denote that, at the point of marital separation, the most turmoil is still experienced in the broken relationship.

Positive Life-Events Dimensions

Age differences were more pronounced when attention turned to positive life events. In general, men and women aged 40 and older experienced fewer positive events at work, in dating and marital activities, in nonfamily relationships, in the personal dimension, and in the overall, summary score of positive experiences. Here again is evidence for an unequal involvement of stressors, with the middle-aged adults being hardest hit. The results suggest that young adults can benefit more than older adults from the separation stage of divorce. For example, men and women aged 40 and older reported experiencing a higher proportion of negative to positive events than did younger respondents. One conclusion is that the breadth of impact is indeed so extensive that it is more appropriate to think of the divorce experience as a "transition" than as a "stressor" or life event. In support of this conclusion, comparisons with subjects in a companion study of normative transitions indicated that divorcing persons were consistently higher in life events across nearly all dimensions, regardless of age or gender (Chiriboga et al., 1991).

Advantages of Life-Events Research

As may be apparent from the preceding sections, life-events research still has valuable contributions to make. The technique is useful for those conducting survey research because of its simplicity of concept and approach. The fact that life-events inventories are readily adapted for special populations is both an advantage and disadvantage: an advantage in allowing greater sensitivity to the study population, a disadvantage in that it creates barriers to generalizing results across studies that use different versions.

Disadvantages of Life-Events Research

Although the SRE and its sophisticated weighting system had much to offer, by the middle to late 1970s several researchers began publishing evidence suggesting that the SRE manifests multiple problems in content validity, predictive validity, and generalizability. For example, many of the items included in the SRE are unlikely to occur in middle-aged and older populations (Ander, Lindstrom, & Tibblin, 1974). The practice of combining positive and negative items into a single Life Change Unit (LCU) score was also questioned, as research demonstrated rather conclusively that positive and negative events had differing implications for psychological well-being (e.g., Chiriboga & Cutler, 1980).

One of the most telling problems with the SRE weighting system was that it yielded results that were correlated in the .70 to .90 range with simple counts of events reported (Chiriboga, 1977; Rahe, 1978). It was also found that the LCU score assigned each event, far from representing a weight generalizable across all sociodemographic groups and even across nations, were significantly different. For example, younger and older subjects in the original sample used by Holmes and Rahe (1967) to arrive at their LCU scores differed in assigned LCU on approximately two thirds of the life events (Masuda & Holmes, 1978).

Life Events: Concluding Thoughts

Despite the problems inherent in the SRE, it continues to be the method of choice for many researchers. When used with younger populations, as in a recent study of herpes simplex among men and women aged 20 to 46 years (VanderPlate, Aral, & Magder, 1988), the SRE may be reasonably appropriate as to content validity and general applicability of weights. When the sample includes individuals at midlife and beyond, problems can accrue. One conclusion that can be reached is that the original SRE, and many other event-oriented instruments as well, may be limited in their applicability to special populations such as the elderly.

STRESSORS OF EVERYDAY LIFE

From the mid-1970s onward, an alternative perspective to life events was adopted, that of everyday stressors or hassles. New instrumentation has included alternative life-events inventories, usually including either an expanded number of items or a different approach to weighting events, and alternatives to life events themselves. The latter approach has focused on measures of conditions such as hassles, and the more durable or chronic stressors. Nonevents and anticipated events have also been suggested as relevant to persons of all ages, and there is evidence that for persons in the middle and later years, stressful experiences happening to one's children and friends played an increasingly important role (Lowenthal et al., 1975).

As a way of trying to understand the significance of these alternatives, they may for simplicity be grouped into three categories: the microlevel, mezzolevel, and macrolevel.

Microlevel Stressors

At what can be called the microlevel, the focus is on the stressors of everyday life. Examples include getting caught in a traffic jam, mislaying your social security check, or even not being able to find your favorite dress just when you are heading off to dinner. By far the most commonly experienced stressors, they are also the least studied. In one early panel investigation, Holmes and Holmes (1970) reported that day-to-day events were associated with minor physical complaints including the common cold. Several more studies conclude that day-to-day hassles are correlated more strongly with physical and psychosocial outcomes than are life events (e.g., Lazarus & Folkman, 1984; Weinberger, Hiner, & Tierney, 1987).

Within the field of gerontology there has been little interest in microlevel stressors until comparatively recently. Current research tends to be dominated by an instrument, the Hassles Scale, developed by Lazarus and colleagues (e.g., Lazarus & Folkman, 1984). An increasing number of alternatives are being developed, however. Zautra, Guarnaccia, Reich, and Dohrenwend (1988), for example, have spent several years developing an alternative approach that is briefer, and possibly more applicable to older populations.

Mezzolevel Stressors

The most studied of the three levels, mezzolevel stressors deal with situations that are less frequent than microlevel stressors, but that generally are more memorable and important. Studies of the more chronic stressors (e.g., Pearlin, 1985) fall into this category. In studies of older populations, mezzolevel stressors have been found to predict all sorts of physical, mental, and social dysfunction—everything, in fact, from coronary heart disease (e.g., Lynch, 1977) to general psychiatric symptomatology (e.g., Chiriboga, 1984; Dohrenwend, 1986) to depression (e.g., Brown, Bifulco, Harris, & Bridge, 1986; Pearlin, 1980).

Chronic Stress as New Interest Area

Although much of the focus in developmental research on stress has been on life events, which tap acute conditions, the more chronic conditions of life have also received attention. According to theorists such as Pearlin (1980) and Pearlin et al. (1981), in fact, chronic stressors may have a greater impact on an individual's functional state than acute stressors—which may seem bad, but whose effects tend to dissipate in time. This is a debatable point because many life events, such as bereavement, are especially devastating to those who experience them. Moreover, life events sometimes chain to other events, over time; hence, supposedly temporary life events may extend in impact for considerable lengths of time.

The bottom line is that life events, as viewed at one point, may in fact lead to repetitive conditions that many researchers would judge to constitute chronic stress. For example, one surprising finding from a 12-year longitudinal study of younger and older adults was that when life events at each of the five contact points were correlated, the magnitude of the correlations approximated those found in personality research (e.g., Chiriboga, 1984). This finding indicated both that life events are not random and that they do indeed chain forward in time.

Macrolevel Stressors

Stressors at the macrolevel are those that impact first on society at large. War in the Middle East, bad economic news, a flurry of near-misses in the air lanes, or a spill of environmentally hazardous materials not only make the headlines, but can create anxiety and a generally heightened sense of distress on the part of the populace. Perhaps the earliest investigation of macrolevel events was conducted inadvertently. In the United States, Norman Bradburn and his colleague David Caplovitz were testing a new morale measure in a series of national probability studies conducted before and after the assassination of President John Kennedy. They found a national increase in the experiencing of negative emotions in the wake of the murder (Bradburn & Caplovitz, 1965).

More recently Harvey Brenner (1985), a sociologist at Johns Hopkins University, has reported a very strong linkage between downturns in the U.S. economy and upturns in admission rates to mental institutions. In part because of findings such as this, gerontologists are now becoming interested in the role of macrolevel events, which are viewed as having the potential for creating not only change in the short run but change that may affect the trajectory of the individual's entire life (e.g., Birren, 1988; Miller, 1980a). Perhaps the best known macrolevel research, however, is Elder's (1974, 1981) qualitative analysis of the long-term impact of the Great Depression, developed on the basis of data from the Institute of Human Development, University of California, Berkeley.

Using as a base the more than 50 years of data collected by the Institute of Human Development, Berkeley, Elder (1981) evaluated the lasting consequences for children of growing up during the Great Depression that occurred in America during the late 1920s and early 1930s. He found that the Great Depression era exerted either a pervasive and long-term impact on the course of adult life or very little, depending on how old the adult was during the early 1930s.

One conclusion that can be drawn from Elder's work, as well as from the writings of authors such as Burke (1984) and Lasch (1984), is that the adult life course is affected by the social and physical environment. In his own treatise on the Great Depression, for example, Burke (1984) has concluded that major social change can lead to an "unsettling" of individuals because it requires change in the customary way of thinking.

Given such evidence, it seems important to begin to develop more refined ways of assessing macrolevel stressors. Knowing more about how events on a world-scale level affect our personal well-being will begin to help us to understand and predict the trajectories of adult life both now and in the future. That is, such work would aid social scientists immeasurably in our efforts to comprehend the ways in which the adult life course is played out.

Example of Research

In aging, as in stress research in general, the least attention seems to have been paid to macrolevel stressors. An exception is Miller's (1980a) early work assessing the impact of exposure to the media. A companion study to the divorce project discussed earlier (Fiske & Chiriboga, 1990) did develop a relevant instrument: the Social Change Scale. The study looked at people at five points during a 12-year period. At the first contact, the sample included high school seniors, newlyweds, middle-aged parents, and people facing retirement. A Social Change Scale was administered at all contacts. As originally developed, it included 10 items. Five were events of the past (the Great Depression, etc.), and five were for the present. The five present conditions, for example, consisted of new ways of completing tasks at work, changing roles of women, changes in rights of minorities, crime in the streets, and changes in the economy and employment. For each item, respondents circled whether it had no, little, moderate, or strong effect on them. At the last session, three new items were added: the international situation, dangers at nuclear plants, and new life-styles.

When we looked at scores from the Social Change Scale, we found that they were significantly associated with psychological symptoms and affect balance among older adults (Chiriboga, 1984; Fiske & Chiriboga, 1985, 1990). The kinds of items endorsed also were of interest. For example, at the fourth contact, somewhat less than a third of the youngest men, now aged 20 to mid-30s, cited changes in rights of minorities and about the same proportion were concerned about new roles for women. Because most of these young men had only recently entered the labor market it seems likely that they felt threatened about potential competition. Youngest women were equally concerned about new roles and crime in the streets. Newlywed men worried about new ways at work and changes in the economy. Their female counterparts cited changing roles of women as well as the economy. The four older groups were less varied in their response: crime on the streets was the big problem, and the proportion singling that item out ranged from two fifths of the oldest women to two thirds of the middle-aged men.

Two years later, changes in the economy and employment were foremost in the minds of the young, ranging from a third or more of the youngest people to well over half of the newlyweds of both sexes. All of the four oldest groups had become even more worried about crime. For example, two fifths of the oldest women cited crime at the fourth interview, but four fifths of them did so at the last one. In fact, most of these women had become more worried about everything.

Advantages of Everyday Approach

Letting go of the Schedule of Recent Events as the standard "tool" of the trade has had the advantage of freeing researchers to explore more innovative and diverse approaches to stress measurement. The active pursuit of alternatives to life-events methodologies has generated a wealth of concepts and instruments designed to assess stressors. The result is that researchers today, whether they are gerontologists or child counselors, have available several options when selecting instruments.

Disadvantages of Everyday Approach

One drawback to the rapid proliferation and evolution of stress indexes during the past decade has been that there are now, in a sense, too many choices. Many of the newer instruments are still in development stage, and the psychometric properties are often poorly described.

A related but perhaps less obvious problem is that many of the existing instruments are undergoing continuous evolution. Although it was not difficult to track changes in the SRE, tracking even the 10 to 15 measures relevant to aging can be difficult. In consequence, those who adopt the instruments are often using instruments that are months to years out of date or are using them in ways that the original authors have now abandoned.

As an example, in the late 1970s Lazarus and his colleagues at University of California, Berkeley, developed several instruments to tap dimensions of stress including measures of hassles and uplifts and coping (e.g., Lazarus & Launier, 1978). Although several of these indexes were modified in later work (e.g., Lazarus & Folkman, 1984), many researchers and practitioners continue to use the original version. Similarly, the geriatric life events inventory developed by Eva Kahana and her colleagues (Kahana, Kiyak & Liang, 1980; Kiyak et al., 1976) has undergone considerable revision since its initial development. Although Kahana (personal communication, June 10, 1988) believes the resulting instruments are much improved, others continue to use an older version that represents work conducted up to 10 years in the past.

Sometimes, of course, it may be necessary to continue using older versions. For example, in longitudinal research in which the focus is on test and retest during considerable periods, the researcher may quite rightly be unwilling to modify or change an instrument. When replicating or expanding on existing research, an investigator may decide to use an older instrument that has been used in the previous work.

Another drawback of investigations conducted under the rubric of the stressors of everyday life model is that one particular instrument is often being advanced, implicitly or explicitly, as the analytic or measurement approach to follow. In part this may reflect the last vestiges of the revolt against the life-event paradigm. There is often an effort made to contrast the efficacy of a new approach, such as hassles (DeLongis et al., 1982) or chronic stressors (e.g., Pearlin et al., 1981) as opposed to traditional life-event measures, as is common with shifting paradigms. Although such studies have clearly illustrated the advantages of using new measurement procedures, what is sometimes lost is that life events, hassles, and the more durable stressors all may play a role in determining the outcome of stress exposure.

Once again, therefore, we find that stress research has not found its particular version of paradise. Currently there exist a host of alternative—and sometimes competing—approaches to defining stressors.

INTEGRATED MODEL OF SOCIAL STRESSORS

Stress research would seem to be entering an age of complexity, one in which the empirical models are not only sophisticated but include multiple approaches to measurement of the stressor component of the stress paradigm. Researchers are beginning to recognize the value of not just one, but many, of the new approaches to stress measurement that have been developed. Increasingly, we are seeing efforts to study people laboring under conditions of severe stress (reflecting the catastrophe model) as well as coping with life events, hassles, and chronic stressors, and interacting with their environments.

Growing Appreciation of Transactionist Perspective

One characteristic of the more integrated approaches to stress research is a recognition that stress exposure does not occur in a vacuum, but is influenced by both the general context, and by continuing transactions between the person and the environment. For some time, stress researchers have recognized that the stress process is one best portrayed not by simple mechanistic models but rather by transactional models. In other words, stress represents a transaction between the individual and the environment. Not only does this point become relevant after exposure to a stressor but indeed it is relevant throughout. For example, several researchers have considered the question of the fit between the individual and the environment. In one early study, Turner (1968) considered whether certain personality styles make for a better fit between older people and an institutional environment. Out of this research came the idea that "grouchy" people may fare better in institutional settings, possibly because, by being more demanding and complaining, their needs are better met.

More recently, Hobfoll (1988) has considered what he terms "ecological congruence." His position is that one must consider the nature of the demands imposed by the environment as well as the real and perceived resources of the individual. Overall, the significance of the person-environment transaction is being emphasized more and more in stress theories and research (e.g., Hobfoll, 1988; Wilson, 1989). Both in studies of extreme trauma (e.g., Wilson, 1989) and of everyday stressors (e.g., Hobfoll, 1988; Lazarus & Folkman, 1984), such transactions are viewed as critical.

Study of Caregiving

The integrative model is illustrated in an ongoing study of adult child caregivers and their dependent parents that is directed by the author. The study represents an attempt to integrate theoretical models drawn from stress research (e.g., Fiske & Chiriboga, 1990; Hobfoll, 1988; Lazarus & Folkman, 1984) with models of social exchange and social justice (e.g., Lerner, Somers, Reid, & Tierney, 1989).

Study participants lived in the Central Valley area of Northern California; they included not only adult child caregivers but also the parent afflicted with Alzheimer's disease as well. The caregivers were drawn from a variety of sources: children of parents who were seeking care in either a university geriatric clinic or a state-funded Alzheimer's Disease Diagnosis and Treatment Center, participants in several local chapters of the Alzheimer's Disease and Related Disorders Association, children of parents institutionalized in approximately 20 skilled and intermediate care nursing facilities, and community center referrals. In all cases, the basic screening requirement was that there be two adult children available for interview and one parent with a probable diagnosis of Alzheimer's disease.

Measurement Issues

Because the caregiver study covered some uncharted territories in the domain of stress, we developed a battery of structured as well as unstructured interview questions. Social stressors, a pivotal variable in the study, were to be looked at as playing potentially a pivotal role in determining both the provision of care and the well-being of caregivers, the parent, and indeed the entire family.

In studying the stress exposure of adult caregiver, one basic decision that had to be reached concerned how broad a range of stressors should be included. We have already seen that stressors are sometimes operationalized as life events, sometimes as more chronic problems such as continuing friction with colleagues at work or the need to provide care to a dependent parent. They may be major events, such as the birth of a child or the death of a spouse, and they may be day-to-day events such as getting tied up in traffic or running out of cereal in the morning. They may even be positive experiences, if these experiences create major change and disequilibrium in the person's life.

Clearly there are a host of stressors that can affect the well-being of caregivers, and these stressors are not necessarily related directly to caregiving. Because of their potential, we included not only stressors specific to caregiving but those of a more general nature, such as work and financial stressors. Measures tapped general life events, hassles, and perceived burden of care; unstructured questions were also included as a check on the content validity of structured instruments.

Additional Measures in Stress Paradigm

Naturally, indicators of stress exposure and perceptions of stress were not the only measures relevant to the stress paradigm. We also included a 56-item modified Ways of Coping Scale (Lazarus & Folkman, 1984); three established indicators of psychological functioning were included in this study (the Bradburn Affect Balance and the Anxiety and Depression subscales from the Hopkins Symptoms Checklist-90), measures of social support and resources, measures of self-concept, assessments by caregivers of parent's premorbid personality, family tensions related to decisions about caring and actual care provision, and so on.

We also included a total score based on the Assistance With Daily Life Scale (AWDLS; alpha = .93); the AWDLS asked adult children how often they assisted their parent with each of 14 activities of daily life. For example, how often did they make telephone calls for the parent, take them to the doctor, help in the preparation of meals, and so on. In each case, an 8-point rating scale was used, where 1 = "never" and 8 = "more than once a day."

Predicting Well-Being of Caregivers

One series of analyses have compared the association of general stressors, versus caregiver-specific stressors, when looking at the well-being of caregivers. We did this by computing hierarchical-set regression analyses for three measures of caregiver well-being: affect balance, anxiety, and depression. In each regression, the variable sets were entered in the following order: (a) basic demographics, (b) parent characteristics, (c) social supports, (d) subjective and objective burden, and (e) events and hassles. The following discussion focuses on findings from the last two sets.

After the contribution of sets a through c were partialed out, we found that affect balance was not predicted by the objective and subjective indexes of burden and did not contribute to morale, either individually or as a set (Chiriboga, Weiler, & Nielsen, 1989). The measures of life events and hassles, entered as the fifth anf final set, did make a contribution, however. In fact, for the regression equation predicting affect balance, the largest contribution came from the general, noncaregiver events and hassles, and not from the indexes focused specifically on caregiver stress and strain. More specifically, fewer work events, work hassles, and hassles in social relationships together accounted for a substantial 17% of the variance in affect balance.

These findings imply that for researchers interested in the morale of caregivers, a focus on predictive indexes such as objective or subjective burden may represent too narrow a view. Researchers and clinicians may in fact be better off examining the overall array of stressors confronting the caregiver who has other worries in addition to the work entailed by the presence of a dependent parent or sibling. At the same time it should also be remembered that the more focused measures also contributed significantly to the prediction of caregiver morale and are certainly worthy of consideration.

A third measure of subjective burden, that of unreasonable parental demands, was also involved in the predictive equation. Although involved only to a minor extent, it is worth noting because in the zero-order correlation there was no relationship. In the context of the other variables, however, a suppressor relationship emerged: caregivers who felt their parent made unreasonable demands were less depressed. One explanation may be that perceiving the parent to be unreasonably demanding makes it easier for caregivers to distance themselves from the situation.

Once again, however, the greatest amount of variance continued to be accounted for by general indexes of stress (Chiriboga et al., 1989). In addition, caregivers with more work events, work hassles, and hassles with social relationships came out as more depressed. One new contributor was spousal hassles: those reporting hassles with their spouse were significantly more depressed.

Importance of Overall Levels of Stress

Overall the findings from the caregiver study point to the value of casting a broad predictive net of stress indexes when studying individuals who may be experiencing stressful lives. Stress situations specific to the caregiving role are clearly not the only situations of importance for the well-being of caregivers; we should remember that caregivers have other roles to play, other lives to lead. When we as researchers step in, and prepare our armamentarium of measurement tools, we often are so focused on the topic of our own interest that we may exclude a wide range of highly relevant variables. To avoid such exclusions, a more integrative approach seems necessary. One approach may be to include both comprehensive or global measures of stress conditions and measures that are specific to the stress context under investigation.

Advantages. An integrated, transactional approach to the study of stress considers the cumulative effects of life events, catastrophe, and everyday stressors in examining the effects of stress on human beings.

Disadvantages. The integrated approach is limited in its utility, in part, because of measurement concerns, particularly as regards a common metric. Additionally, the complexity of the model requires an equally complex analytical technique.

DISCUSSION

As the field of stress research reaches toward a more integrative approach to modeling the stressor side of the stress-response continuum, comparative evaluations of the adequacy of existing instruments may receive an increasing priority. As gerontologists we may also be interested in whether certain of the measurement approaches are more relevant to older populations than others. Perhaps more important is that we continue to explore the multiple ways in which stressors of different shapes and sizes interact with each other.

Need for Comprehensive Stress Batteries

Gerontologists currently have a wide array of stress-measurement tools to pick from, and are creating more and more each year. Perhaps it is time to consider the virtues of the most promising, or at least weigh the strong and weak points, of measures from the microlevels, mezzolevels, and macrolevels of stress. The intent would not necessarily be to select the single best instrument, because there does not seem to be any single instrument that adequately captures the variance posed by the stressor construct. Rather, the intent might be to develop a comprehensive battery that taps at least the more general sorts of stressors to which individuals may be exposed.

If generally accepted, such a comprehensive battery could serve as a solution to the problem posed by the multiplicity of available instruments. It might be used as a stand-alone instrument, or in conjunction with instruments designed to assess particular stress conditions in more depth: rape, exposure to natural disasters, unemployment, caregiving, and so on.

To create such a battery, it would obviously be necessary to evaluate the psychometric properties of instruments. Here some form of consensus-building procedure would be mandatory. A less obvious need is to gain some sense of how measures from the various levels or domains of stress interrelate. For example, what is the relationship of life events to chronic conditions? It has already been noted that correlations over time of life events are often relatively strong (Fiske & Chiriboga, 1990). In other words, life events are not necessarily incidents that happen by chance: there may be a repetition of events over time. The question then becomes how and when do life events become chronic in nature, and vice versa, and do we really need measures of both?

Integration of Stress Measures

Regardless of whether there is a move toward the development of a standard and accepted battery of general stress indicators, more and more researchers are integrating stress measures of different levels and types in their studies. This trend will undoubtedly lead to advances in our understanding of the relationship of stressors not only with outcomes but with other stressors. We may find, for example, that stressors from one domain are not only somewhat related but may act as potentiators and catalysts. Having a heavy dose of macrolevel or mezzolevel stressors may lead to a situation in which the individual exhibits an exacerbated impact to what would seem to be a minor life event or day-to-day hassle. In the divorce study, for example, we found evidence of an accumulation of life events in all domains of life (Chiriboga et al., 1991). This phenomenon we labeled the "camel's back syndrome," because at a certain point any additional stress appeared to create a greater than predictable response.

Given what appears to be the emergence of a more integrated model of stress research, the 1990s may witness a blending of the previous approaches. One point to reemphasize is that none of the four models of stress that have been discussed is in fact mutually exclusive. In many ways, we are now coming full circle in stress research, and once again using samples of people who are obviously under duress. This time around, however, we can employ indexes of the specific stress context as well as the general levels of stress exposure instead of merely assuming that individuals are all equally stressed. Such a strategy has certain advantages over those used in earlier approaches to catastrophe research. Overall, then, the conclusion one may draw from this brief review is that stress researchers may have lost Paradise several times, but they very well may be in the process of creating a new one.

REFERENCES

Aldrich, C. K., & Mendkoff, E. (1963). Relocation of the aged and disabled: A mortality study. *Journal of the American Geriatric Society, 11*, 185–194.

Aldwin, C. M., & Revenson, T. A. (1987). Does coping help? A reexamination of the relation between coping and mental health. *Journal of Personality and Social Psychology, 53*, 337–348.

American Psychiatric Association. (1987). *Diagnostic and statistical manual of mental disorders* (3rd ed.). Washington, DC: Author.

Amster, L. E., & Krauss, H. H. (1974). The relationship between life events and mental deterioration in old age. *International Journal of Aging and Human Development, 5*, 51–55.

Ander, S., Lindstrom, B., & Tibblin, G. (1974). Life changes in random samples of middle-aged men. In E. K. Gunderson & R. H. Rahe (Eds.), *Life stress and illness* (pp. 121–124). Springfield, IL: Charles C Thomas.

Antonovsky, A., Leibowitz, U., Smith, H. A., Medalie, J. M., Balogh, M., Kats, R., Halpern, L., & Alter, M. (1965). Epidemiologic study of multiple sclerosis in Israel: I. An overall review of methods and findings. *Archives of Neurology, 13,* 183–193.

Baum, A. (1987). Toxins, technology and natural disasters. In G. R. VandenBos & B. K. Bryant (Eds.), *Cataclysms, crises, and catastrophes: Psychology in action* (pp. 5–53). Washington, DC: American Psychological Association.

Birren, J. E. (1988). A contribution to the theory of the psychology of aging: As a counterpart of development. In J. E. Birren & V. L. Bengtson (Eds.), *Emergent theories of aging* (pp. 153–176). New York: Springer.

Bradburn, N., & Caplovitz, D. (1965). *Reports on happiness: A pilot study of behavior related to mental health.* Chicago: Aldine.

Brenner, M. H. (1985). Economic change and the suicide rate: A population model including loss, separation, illness, and alcohol consumption. In M. R. Zales (Ed.), *Stress in health alnd disease* (pp. 160–185). New York: Brunner/Mazel.

Breuer, J., & Freud, S. (1955). *The standard edition of the complete psychological works of Sigmund Freud* (Vol. 2). London: Hogarth Press.

Brody, E. M. (1989). The family at risk. In E. Light & B. D. Lebowitz (Eds.), *Alzheimer's disease treatment and family stress: Directions for research* (DHHS Publication No. ADM 89-1569, pp. 2–49). Washington, DC: U.S. Government Printing Office.

Brown, G. W., Bifulco, A., Harris, T., & Bridge, L. (1986). Life stress, chronic subclinical symptoms and vulnerability to clinical depression. *Journal of Affective Disorders, 11,* 1–119.

Burke, K. (1984). *Permanence and change* (3rd ed.). Los Angeles: University of California Press.

Chiriboga, D. A. (1972). *The prediction of relocation stress among the aged: A comparative study.* Unpublished doctoral dissertation, University of Chicago.

Chiriboga, D. A. (1977). Life event weighting systems: A comparative analysis. *Journal of Psychosomatic Research, 21,* 415–422.

Chiriboga, D. A. (1984). Social stressors as antecedents of change. *Journal of Gerontology, 39,* 468–477.

Chiriboga, D. A., & Bailey, J. T. (1989). Burnout and coping among hospital nurses: Research and guidelines for action. In B. Riegel & D. Ehrenreich (Eds.), *Psychological aspects of critical care nursing* (pp. 295–323). Rockville, MD: Aspen.

Chiriboga, D. A., Catron, L. S., & Associates (1991). *Divorce: Crisis, challenge or relief?* New York: New York University Press.

Chiriboga, D. A., & Cutler, L. (1980). Stress and adaptation: Life span perspectives. In L. W. Poon (Ed.), *Aging in the 1980s: Psychological issues* (pp. 347–362). Washington, DC: American Psychological Association.

Chiriboga, D. A., & Dean, H. (1978). Dimensions of stress: Perspectives from a longitudinal study. *Journal of Psychosomatic Research, 22,* 47–55.

Chiriboga, D. A., Weiler, P. G., & Nielsen, K. (1989). The stress of caregivers. *Journal of Applied Social Sciences, 13,* 118–141.

Cohen, C. I., Teresi, J., & Holmes, D. (1985). Social networks, stress, and physical health: A longitudinal study of an inner-city elderly population. *Journal of Gerontology, 40,* 478–486.

Cohen, F., & Lazarus, R. S. (1973). Active coping processes, coping dispositions, and recovery from surgery. *Psychosomatic Medicine, 35,* 375–389.

Deimling, G. T., Bass, D. M., Townsend, A. L., & Noelker, L. S. (1989). Care-related stress: A comparison of spouse and adult-child caregivers in shared and separate households. *Journal of Aging and Health, 1,* 67–82.

DeLongis, A., Coyne, J. C., Dakof, G., Folkman, S., & Lazarus, R. S. (1982). Relationship of daily hassles, uplifts, and major life events to health status. *Health Psychology, 1,* 119–136.

Dohrenwend, B. P. (1986). Note on a program of research on alternative social psychological models of relationships between life stress and psychopathology. In M. H. Appley & R. Trumbull (Eds.), *Dynamics of stress: Physiological, psychological and social perspectives* (pp. 283–293). New York: Plenum.

Dohrenwend, B. S., Krasnoff, L., Askenasy, A., & Dohrenwend, B. P. (1978). Exemplification of a method for scaling life events: The PERI Life Events Scale. *Journal of Health and Social Behavior, 19,* 205–229.

Dunkel-Schetter, C. (1984). Social support and cancer: Findings based on patient interviews and their implications. *Journal of Social Issues, 40,* 77–98.

Elder, G. H., Jr. (1974). *Children of the Great Depression: Social change in life experience.* Chicago: University of Chicago Press.

Elder, G. H., Jr. (1981). Social history and life experience. In D. H. Eichorn, J. A. Clausen, N. Haan, M. P. Honzik, & P. H. Mussen (Eds.), *Present and past in middle life* (pp. 3–31). New York: Academic Press.

Fiske, M., & Chiriboga, D. A. (1985). The interweaving of societal and personal change in adulthood. In J. M. A. Munnichs, P. Mussen, E. Olbrich, & P. G. Coleman (Eds.), *Life-span and change in a gerontological perspective* (pp. 177–209). Orlando: Academic Press.

Fiske, M., & Chiriboga, D. A. (1990). *Change and continuity in adult life.* San Francisco: Jossey-Bass.

Friedsam, H. J. (1960). Older persons as disaster casualties. *Journal of Health and Human Behavior, 1*, 269–273.

Golan, N. (1978). *Treatment in crisis situations.* New York: Free Press.

Grinker, R. R., & Spiegel, J. P. (1963). *Men under stress.* New York: McGraw-Hill.

Gutmann, D. L. (1964). An exploration of ego configurations in middle and later life. In B. L. Neugarten & Associates (Eds.), *Personality in middle and Later Life* (pp. 114–148). New York: Atherton.

Gutmann, D. L. (1985). The parental imperative revisited. In J. Meacham (Ed.), *Family and individual development* (pp. 31–60). Basel: Karger.

Hobfoll, S. E. (1988). *The ecology of stress.* New York: Hemisphere.

Holmes, T. S., & Holmes, T. H. (1970). Short-term intrusions into the life-style routine. *Journal of Psychosomatic Research, 14*, 121–132.

Holmes, T., & Rahe, R. (1967). The social readjustment rating scale. *Journal of Psychosomatic Research, 11*, 213–218.

Horowitz, M. J. (1986). *Stress response syndromes* (2nd ed.). New Jersey: Jason Aronson.

Horowitz, M. J., & Wilner, N. (1980). Life events, stress, and coping. In L. W. Poon (Ed.), *Aging in the 1980s: Psychological issues* (pp. 363–374). Washington, DC: American Psychological Association.

Hunter, E. J. (1988). The psychological effects of being a prisoner of war. In J. P. Wilson, Z. Harel, & B. Kahana (Eds.), *Human adaptation to extreme stress: From the Holocaust to Vietnam* (pp. 157–170). New York: Plenum.

Janis, J. (1958). *Psychological stress: Psychoanalytic and behavioral studies of surgical patients.* New York: Wiley & Sons.

Kahana, B., Harel, Z., & Kahana, E. (1988). Predictors of psychological well-being among survivors of the Holocaust. In J. P. Wilson, Z. Harel, & B. Kahana (Eds.), *Human adaptation in extreme stress: From the Holocaust to Vietnam* (pp. 55–79). New York: Plenum.

Kahana, E. F., Kahana, B., & Young, R. (1987). Influences of diverse stress on health and well-being of community aged. In A. M. Fowler (Ed.), *Post traumatic stress: The healing journey.* Washington DC: Veterans Administration.

Kahana, E., Kiyak, A., & Liang, J. (1980). Menopause in the context of other life events. In A. Dann, E. Graham, & C. Beecher (Eds.), *The menstrual cycle* (pp. 167–178). New York: Springer.

Kemeny, M. E., Cohen, F., Zegans, L. S., & Conant, M. A. (1989). Psychological and immunological predictors of genital herpes recurrence. *Psychosomatic Medicine, 51*, 195–208.

Kiyak, A., Liang, J., & Kahana, E. (1976, August). *A methodological inquiry into the schedule of recent life events.* Paper presented at the meeting of the American Psychological Association, Washington, DC.

Krause, N. (1986a). Life stress as a correlate of depression among older adults. *Psychiatry Research, 18,* 227–237.

Krause, N. (1986b). Stress and coping: Reconceptualizing the role of locus of control beliefs. *Journal of Gerontology, 41,* 617–622.

Kubler-Ross, E. (1969). *On death and dying.* New York: Macmillan.

Lasch, C. (1984). *The minimal self.* New York: Norton.

Lazarus, R. S., & Folkman, S. (1984). *Stress, appraisal and coping.* New York: Springer.

Lazarus, R. S., & Launier, R. (1978). Stress-related transactions between person and environment. In L. A. Pervin & M. Lewis (Eds.), *Perspectives in interaction psychology* (pp. 287–327). New York: Plenum.

Lerner, M. J., Somers, D. G., Reid, D. W., Tierney, M. C. (1989). A social dilemma: Egocentrically-biased cognitions among filial caregivers. In S. Spacapan & S. Oskamp (Eds.), *The social psychology of aging: Claremont symposium on applied social psychology* (pp. 53–80). Beverly Hills: Sage.

Lewinsohn, P. M., & MacPhillamy, D. J. (1974). The relationship between age and engagement in pleasant activities. *Journal of Gerontology, 29,* 290–294.

Lewinsohn, P. M., Mermelstein, R. M., Alexander, C., & MacPhillamy, D. J. (1985). The Unpleasant Events Schedule: A scale for the measurement of aversive events. *Journal of Clinical Psychology, 41,* 483–498.

Lewinsohn, P. M., & Talkington, J. (1979). Studies on the measurement of unpleasant events and relations with depression. *Applied Psychological Measurement, 3,* 83–101.

Lieberman, M. A., Prock, V. N., & Tobin, S. S. (1968). Psychological effects of institutionalization. *Journal of Gerontology, 23,* 343–353.

Lindemann, E. (1944). Symptomatology and management of acute grief. *American Journal of Psychiatry, 101,* 141–148.

Lowenthal, M. F., Berkman, P. L., & Associates. (1967). *Aging and mental disorder in San Francisco: A social psychiatric study.* San Francisco: Jossey-Bass.

Lowenthal, M. F., Thurnher, M., & Chiriboga, D. A. (1975). *Four Stages of Life.* San Francisco: Jossey-Bass.

Lynch, J. J. (1977). *The broken heart: The medical consequences of loneliness.* New York: Basic Books.

Masuda, M., & Holmes, T. H. (1978). Life events: Perceptions and frequencies. *Psychosomatic Medicine, 40,* 236–261.

Mensh, I. N. (1983). A study of a stress questionnaire: The later years. *Internat”ional Journal of Aging & Human Development, 16,* 201–207.

Miller, F. T. (1980a). Measurement and monitoring of stress in communities. In L. W. Poon (Ed.), *Aging in the 1980s: Psychological issues* (pp. 383–388). Washington, DC: American Psychological Association.

Miller, S. M. (1980b). When is a little knowledge a dangerous thing? Coping with stressful life events by monitoring vs. blunting. In S. Levine & H. Ursine (Eds.), Coping and health (pp. 145–169). New York: Plenum.

Miller, S. M. (in press). Monitors and blunters. In L. Montada, S.-H. Filipp, & M. Lerner. Life crises and experiences of loss in adulthood. New York: Plenum.

Murrell, S. A., Norris, F. H., & Grote, C. (1987). Life events in older adults. In L. H. Cohen (Ed.), Life events and psychological functioning: Theoretical and methodological issues (pp. 96–122). Beverly Hills: Sage.

Murrell, S. A., Norris, F. H., & Hutchins, G. L. (1984). Distribution and desirability of life events in older adults: Population and policy implications. Journal of Community Psychology, 12, 301–311.

Noshpitz, J. D., & Coddington, R. D. (Eds.). (1990). Stressors and the adjustment disorders. Somerset, NJ: Wiley & Sons.

Pearlin, L. I. (1980). Life strains and psychological distress among adults. In N. J. Smelser & E. H. Erikson (Eds.), Themes of work and love in adulthood (pp. 174–192). Cambridge, MA: Harvard University Press.

Pearlin, L. I. (1985). Life strains and psychological distress among adults. In A. Monat & R. S. Lazarus (Eds.), Stress and coping: An anthology (2nd ed., pp. 192–207). New York: Columbia University Press.

Pearlin, L. I., Menaghan, E. G., Lieberman, M. A., & Mullan, J. T. (1981). The stress process. Journal of Health and Social Behavior, 22, 337–356.

Pearlin, L. I., & Schooler, C. (1978). The structure of coping. Journal of Health and Social Behavior, 19, 2–21.

Phifer, J. F. (1990). Psychological distress and somatic symptoms after natural disaster: Differential vulnerability among older adults. Psychology and Aging, 5, 412–420.

Pollack, H. M. (1925). What happens to patients during the first year of hospital life? Albany, NY: State Hospital Commission.

Pruchno, R. A., & Resch, N. L. (1989). Husbands and wives as caregivers: Antecedents of depression and burden. The Gerontologist, 29, 159–165.

Quayhagen, M., & Chiriboga, D. A. (1976). Geriatric coping scales: Potentials and problems. Paper presented at the 29th annual scientific meeting of the Gerontology Society, New York.

Rahe, R. H. (1978). Life change measurement clarification. Psychosomatic Medicine, 40, 95–98.

Selye, H. The stress of life. (1956). New York: McGraw-Hill.

Singer, E. (1988). Delay behavior among women with breast symptoms. In T. M. Field, P. M. McCabe, & N. Schneiderman (Eds.), Stress and coping across development (pp. 163–188). Hillsdale, NJ: Erlbaum.

Taylor, S. E., & Dakof, G. A. (1988). Social support and the cancer patient. In S. Spacapan & S. Oskamp (Eds.), The social psychology of health (pp. 95–116). Beverly Hills: Sage.

Teri, L., & Lewinsohn, P. (1982). Modification of the pleasant and unpleasant events schedules for use with the elderly. *Journal of Consulting and Clinical Psychology, 50,* 444–445.

Tobin, S. S., & Lieberman, M. A. (1976). *Last home for the aged.* San Francisco: Jossey-Bass.

Tryon, R. C., & Bailey, D. E. (1970). *Cluster analysis.* New York: McGraw-Hill.

Turner, B. F. (1968). *Psychological predictors of adaptation to the distress of institutionalization in the aged.* Unpublished doctoral dissertation, University of Chicago.

Tyhurst, J. S. (1957). Psychological and social aspects of civilian disaster. *Canadian Medical Association Journal, 76,* 385–393.

VanderPlate, C., Aral, S. O., & Magder, L. (1988). The relationship among genital herpes simplex virus, stress and social support. *Health Psychology, 7,* 159–168.

Weinberger, M., Hiner, S. L., & Tierney, W. M. (1987). In support of hassles as a measure of stress in predicting health outcomes. *Journal of Behavioral Medicine, 10,* 19–31.

Wilson, J. P. (1989). *Trauma, transformation, and healing: An integrative approach to theory, research, and post-traumatic therapy.* New York: Brunner/Mazel.

Wortman, C. B., & Silver, R. C. (1987). Coping with irrevocable loss. In G. R. VandenBos & B. K. Bryant (Eds.), *Cataclysms, crises, and catastrophes: Psychology in action* (pp. 185–235). Washington, DC: American Psychological Association.

Zautra, A. J., Guarnaccia, C. A., Reich, J. W., & Dohrenwend, B. P. (1988). The contribution of small events to stress and distress. In L. H. Cohen (Ed.), *Life events and psychological functioning: Theoretical and methodological issues* (pp. 123–148). Beverly Hills: Sage.

3

Social Support Processes in Health and Effective Functioning of the Elderly

James S. Jackson and Toni C. Antonucci

Since the initial clinical observations (e.g., Cassel, 1976; Cobb, 1976) the concept of, and research on, social support has become ubiquitous (House, Umberson, & Landis, 1988), but particularly so in the social gerontological literature (Antonucci, 1990). The construct and the attendant concerns with stress and coping are of important theoretical, clinical, and public policy concern (Antonucci & Jackson, 1987; Sarason, Sarason, & Pierce, 1990). It is the importance of the social support construct in all three arenas that has contributed not only to the profusion of work in the area, but also to much of the confusion and lack of clarity in the literature. Theoreticians (e.g., Litwak, 1985) and researchers in the field (e.g., House et al., 1988) have been concerned with how social and psychological stress induced from environmental and internal sources are mediated by the individual embedded within personal networks. Historically, interest in this area stemmed from some of the earliest writings on social integration and social isolation (House et al., 1988) as well as the concerns with the nature and process of stress and coping as adaptive responses (Pearlin, 1989).

In social gerontology a long-standing interest in adjustment, reactions to loss, and life transitions make the social support construct of central importance (Antonucci, 1990; Stephens, Crowther, Hobfoll, & Tennenbaum, 1990). A multitude of disciplines, and particularly sociology (Huber & Spitze, 1988), have also had long-standing concern with how the family system operates in concert with other institutions to provide environmental contexts for optimal development (Boissevain, 1974; Bott, 1957; Huber & Spitze, 1988). Recently many scholars have suggested the need to understand social support within an individual life-course framework that emphasizes early social and family development in attachment with later development in adolescence and adulthood (Ishii-Kuntz & Seccombe, 1989; Kreppner, 1989). Theoretically, this more recent view places social support squarely within the socialization and intrapersonal and interpersonal processes domain (Antonucci & Jackson, 1987; House et al., 1988), one that we believe offers the most fruitful scientific potential.

The graying of America is occurring with relative rapidity, portending significant strains on an already burdened and expensive health care delivery system (Jackson, 1988; Stephens et al., 1990). It is becoming apparent that the nation will not be able to afford both continued increases in the level of coverage and rising numbers of individuals needing and desiring services. Some estimates indicate that at current rates of increase that health care costs will so dominate the gross national product that the nation will have no discretionary resources for addressing other pressing needs. In fact, it has been the health concerns that have generated much of the current debate about "greedy geezers" and intergenerational equity. Thus, it is probable that the increasing numbers of older individuals in need of care are straining the nation's capacity to care for them (Soldo & Manton, 1985). In addition to acute care, chronic care arising from long-term disability also raises serious issues. Some projections indicate that the United States will suffer a serious deficiency in long-term care facilities during the next decade or so, given the projections in the number of frail elderly (Jackson, Antonucci, & Gibson, 1990). When combined with questionable practices and policies, with the lack of enforceable regulations or oversight in long-term care facilities, a growing concern about the distribution of tax dollars, and a growing lack of private insurance among the elderly, the opportunity for providing appropriate care for the increasingly frail very old, and thus potentially dependent, population is problematic (Rathbone-McCuan,

Hooyman, & Fortune, 1985). These problems are exacerbated because the fastest growing older populations are among racial and ethnic minorities, groups whose health care needs, because of lifetimes of neglect, may prove to be even more expensive to address than individuals in the general population (Jackson et al., 1990; Lubben & Becerra, 1987).

Many have suggested that the family is the logical and most reasonable source of care, perhaps even preferable to the formal system (Antonucci, 1989). The combination of a decrease in average family size during several decades and the move toward increasingly disparate extended family systems, however, has led to a call for formal and friend networks to meet the care needs of the elderly (Ferraro, Mutran, & Barresi, 1984; Litwak, 1985; Stephens et al., 1990). Although many note the historical role of the family in caring for dependent family members in the United States, a practice still common in other parts of the world, the change in the nature of the American family system and the increased mobility of the population, make the family a less than assured alternative to formal care.

Thus, the work on social support, especially among older populations, shows a unique confluence of interests including theoretical and scientific work on the sociology of the family, the role of stress, and the nature of small-group interaction (Hobfoll & Freedy, 1990; Pearlin, Mullan, Semple, & Skaff, 1990). Clinically, concern with health and effective functioning in the face of rising costs and decreased resources makes the role of family and friend support of critical importance in the course and recovery from illness and disability. Finally, dealing with rising health care costs and trade-offs between a healthy citizenry and competing costs for rebuilding the physical infrastructure, revitalizing an antiquated educational system, and providing opportunities directed largely at the young pose important public policy dilemmas for the nature of family assistance plans and family support programs (e.g., Kiesler, 1985).

The positive role of family and friends in the promotion of health and the prevention of illness are areas that demand the focus of scientists, clinical practitioners, and policy makers (Ferraro et al., 1984). As would be expected within the last two decades, and especially the last 5 to 10 years, the amount of research loosely labeled social support has virtually exploded. In part, this is due not only to the colloquial appeal and topical importance of the social support concept, but also to the fact that the construct and its implications cut across scientific, clinical, and public policy lines.

Popular interest and concern with social support, however, have also contributed to problems in scientific research. In general, researchers have been inconsistent and nonspecific in both the definition and measurement of social support (Antonucci, 1985b; Berkman, 1984; House & Kahn, 1985). Because of its cross-cutting appeal, the term *social support* has not been rigorously and consistently defined. In some cases, researchers have simply measured the existence of social relationships such as marriage, friendships, and family ties, whereas others have actually assessed the quantity and quality of these relationships. The lack of clarity in conceptualization and measurement has been the single greatest failing in interpreting the vast array of research findings in this field. This problem has been even more pronounced in social gerontology because of the immediate and pressing clinical and public policy implications. The lack of agreement and uniformity of definitional, measurement, and methodological approaches have created many problems in interpreting the research literature.

Another problem is that the concept is of interest to research investigators from a variety of disciplines—for example, anthropology, medical sciences, psychology, nursing, sociology, and social work (Antonucci & Jackson, 1987). Based on different historical traditions, methodologies, and theoretical frameworks, it is understandable why scientific approaches lack uniformity. Often different disciplines approach the study of social support to the exclusion of relevant findings from other scientific areas.

In summary, because of the confluence of scientific, clinical, and public policy interests, as well as different disciplinary traditions, the literature has seen a profusion of research on social support during the last two decades. Most recent thinking on the subject views social support within the domain of interpersonal processes and attempts to understand the nature of socially supportive relationships and their consequences on individuals and groups within an individual life-course framework (Antonucci, 1990; House et al., 1988). Many recent reviews of the social support literature relevant to a social-gerontological focus now exist (Antonucci, 1990; Berkman, 1984; Brownell & Shumaker, 1984; Cohen & Wills, 1985; House et al., 1988; Kessler, Price, & Wortman, 1985). Thus, it is not our intention to provide an encyclopedic review of the social support literature. It is our purpose, however, to review a few criticial conceptual and methodological issues relevant to understanding the nature of social support in the health and effective functioning of the elderly. We are particularly concerned with the directions future research may take to inform clinical and public policy decisions. We are concerned with the research that is needed to advance our understanding of the nature and function of social support within an interpersonal, social relationship framework (Coyne & DeLongis, 1986). We provide a brief review of the research and literature that suggests a relationship between social support, and health and effective functioning among aging individuals. We then briefly review some of the possible mechanisms that may undergird and contribute to our understanding of how socially supportive behaviors operate to affect health and effective functioning. Special attention is given to the literature on control, personal efficacy, and related motivational constructs (e.g., Lee & Shehan, 1989). We believe that this work may provide a possible theoretical framework for an interpersonal attribution model that is proposed as one possible mechanism through which social support affects health and well-being (Antonucci & Jackson, 1987; Brehm, 1984; Krause & Keith, 1989). Finally, we explore some of the clinical and public policy implications of the role of social support in the lives of the elderly.

OVERVIEW OF SOCIAL SUPPORT FINDINGS

Definitions of Stress, Coping, and Social Support

We noted earlier the problems with defining constructs related to social support in elderly populations. Both elderly individuals and the later life families in which they are enmeshed often have sources of stress unlike those associated with individuals in earlier life-cycle stages (Brubaker, 1990). The nature of intergenerational relationships, financial difficulties, safety concerns, and declining health compared with earlier points in the life-span are all sources of stress and strain; although these difficulties are not unique to the elderly, they may be perceived and acted upon in unique ways (Brubaker, 1990; Dean, Kolody, Wood, & Ensel, 1989; Morgan, 1988).

Various definitions and ways of measuring social support among the elderly have been proposed. Although they differ greatly in terms of specifics, and thus the manner in which support is measured, basically most definitions have involved the exchange or provision of supportive behaviors. House and Kahn (1985) noted that three basic approaches exist: (a) measures of the existence, quantity, and type of social relationships; (b) measures of network structure; and (c) functional measures of the quality and content of relationships. Dean et al. (1989) suggested that much of the research in this area has failed to assess quality and content of social relationships in the elderly. In their study they found that quality and content of relationships was a multidimensional construct consisting of caring and concern, social integration, and love and affection. Perhaps most important, they found that different dimensions showed almost opposite relationships to depressive symptoms. For example, they speculated that the positive relationship between depressive symptoms and instrumental support and the slight negative relationship to expressive support may have been due to excessive strains on the support network, a finding confirmed by other work (Coyne, Ellard, & Smith, 1990). Conversely, those showing poor health may have greater need for tangible help and less need for expressive forms of support. Both their study and recent theorizing (Sarason et al., 1990) all point to the important role that expectations for support play. Elders' experience with both interpersonal relationships and support exchanges during the life course appear to play a major role in later life in dictating responses to those providing help sources in the face of environmental stressors and disability (Antonucci & Jackson, 1987). We note that the lack of longitudinal research makes it difficult to assess the few life-course models of support provision that do exist (e.g., Litwak, 1985).

Several researchers have outlined the need for more systematic investigation of the definition and measurement of social support (Antonucci & Depner, 1982; Depner, Wethington, & Ingersoll-Dayton, 1984; Gottlieb, 1981; House & Kahn, 1985; Kasl & Berkman, 1981; Mermelstein, Cohen, & Lichtenstein, 1986; Sarason & Sarason, 1985). Most have concluded that social support is a multidimensional construct, especially among the elderly (Dean et al., 1989), and that its particular research and clinical use must be specified more carefully and critically in the future. We have noted earlier that some of the issues that require further specification include the type of supports assessed (e.g., aid, affect, and affirmation); the source of supports (e.g., family, friends, and neighbors); and the recipient's as well as the provider's assessment of the support (e.g., does the recipient of the aid feel aided or smothered?). We can add to this brief list the need for further multidimensional specification, because both continuity and change in the nature of socially supportive relationships and behavior have been noted in elderly individuals as they age (e.g., Field & Minkler, 1988). As noted earlier, Dean et al. (1989) have reported differential relationships to health among ostensibly different dimensions of social support. The lack of prior specification of the definition and measurement may account for some of the oppositional findings in the literature regarding the degree of effects on health and effective functioning in the amount and type of support provided in elderly populations.

Although we view the definition and measurement of social support to be a major aspect of increased understanding of why and how socially supportive behaviors have their effects, several other issues are also of importance. Among these are issues related to quantity versus quality of support, source of support, reciprocity in support, and life-course perspectives on support. First, however, we turn to a brief review of the literature that suggests a relationship between social supportive behaviors, and health and effective functioning in older age.

Health and Effective Functioning

Even though there has been much confusion regarding the definition and measurement of social support, a wide body of literature suggests that social support plays both a positive stress-buffering and main effect (or insulating) role in the health of the elderly (Antonucci, 1990). Numerous studies have documented the positive role of social support in morbidity and mortality, from the now seminal Alameda County study (Berkman & Syme, 1979), which showed a positive association between the existence of social interactions and later survival (e.g., Blazer, 1982; House, Robbins, & Metzner, 1982) to recent studies (e.g., Haug, Breslau, & Folmar, 1989; Revicki & Mitchell, 1990) that document a positive role of socially supportive relationships on emotional health. Significant positive relationships have been found for coronary heart disease (Antonucci & Johnson, in press); decreased hospitalization (Wan & Weissert, 1981); life satisfaction and morale; postponement of need for institutionalization; and decreased need for social and formal services (Antonucci & Jackson, 1987).

There appears to be little question that social supportive behaviors have positive effects on a wide variety of health and well-being measures in the elderly (Seeman & Berkman, 1988). Several questions, however, have been raised about methodological problems in many of the relationships (e.g., Coyne & Bolger, 1990) as well as problems in the stress-support model in adequately explaining the nature of supportive effects (e.g., negative support) or providing an adequate explanatory framework for understanding how socially supportive behaviors might have their effects (Antonucci & Jackson, 1987; Coyne & Bolger, 1990; Coyne & Downey, 1991).

One area of investigation of processes underlying the manner in which social support is effective has been research on the effects of social relationships on immunological functioning (Ader & Cohen, 1984; Jemmott & Locke, 1984). An extensive amount of research has demonstrated a relationship between psychological stress and physiological strain (e.g., French, 1974). Kiecolt-Glaser et al. (1985) demonstrated that self-reported loneliness was related to higher cortisol levels and lower levels of immunocompetence. Although much of this research has been done on relatively young populations, Kiecolt-Glaser et al. (1985) found that cellular immunocompetence in geriatric populations could be enhanced through psychosocial interventions. Much more research is needed to understand how social and psychological processes may influence physiological functioning, especially immune functioning. We have speculated that social support may have more generalized effects on neuroimmunological systems that in turn effect other biological systems (Antonucci & Jackson, 1987). This is purely conjecture and much more research is needed.

If social support does have effects on immune functioning, however, decreased responsiveness (or changes in responsiveness more generally) in these physiological systems with increased age may suggest that different quantities or types of support may become relevant and perhaps more effective at upper ends of the life course. At any rate, the data appear incontrovertible that some aspects of supportive social relationships have positive effects on such divergent aspects of health and well-being in the elderly as psychopathology, morale, cognitive functioning, hospitalization, long-term care, cardiovascular disease, measures of physiological strain, and even mortality. What is not clear is "how" social support elicits these effects and how universal these effects may be on different outcomes in different age and demographic groups or how they influence the individual over the life-span.

Quality Versus Quantity of Support

In earlier work (Antonucci, 1985b, 1990; Antonucci & Jackson, 1987) we noted that the effects of the confidant relationship and the relative importance of quality versus quantity of exchanges in supportive relationships have been demonstrated. Several studies have clearly shown the important role of the presence of a confidant in increasing the well-being and ameliorating depression among older people (Chappell, 1983; Lowenthal & Haven, 1968; Strain & Chappell, 1982). Some research suggests that socially supportive behaviors from nonfamily may be more influential in the quality of life and effective functioning than the quantity of interactions with either family or friends. This work is consistent with recent reports that emphasize the important role that perceived or subjectively evaluated support may play over the more objectively defined amounts of support or exchanges given (Sarason et al., 1990; Ward, Sherman, & LaGory, 1984).

Some earlier studies have found subjective quality of social support to be a better indicator of life satisfaction than quantity of social support (Duff & Hong, 1982), and that the quality of support is more effective in times of crisis than quantity of support (Field & Minkler, 1988, Porritt, 1979). Conversely, Heller and Mansbach (1984) reported that in elderly women both quality and quantity of support are important. McFarlane, Norman, Streiner, and Roy (1984) using a nonrandom sample of Canadian Family Practice patients found that patients reporting smaller networks felt that their networks were more helpful than patients who reported larger networks.

Other researchers, however, have suggested the presence of too small a network can unnecessarily strain support providers (Cohen & Rajkowski, 1982; Felton, Lehmann, Adler, & Burgio, 1981; Jones, 1981; Levitt, Antonucci, Clark, Rotton, & Finley, 1985). Coyne & Gotlib (1983) reported that a negative relationship may exist between depression and social support, particularly from family members. As has been suggested in the work on caretaker burden, the problems and difficulties of caring for a depressed person appear to lead some support providers to be less supportive. Empirical research focusing on the networks of mentally ill patients support this type of theorizing (e.g., Coyne & Downey, 1991; D'Augelli, 1983; Greenblatt, Becerra, & Serafetinides, 1982).

Sources of Support

Another important issue that has recently received attention is how source of support, especially friends versus family, influence the expression and receipt of support and their effects on health and well-being (e.g., Beigel, 1985; Crohan & Antonucci, 1989). Taylor (1985) has demonstrated, at least among the black elderly, that sources of support from friends, kin, and church members provide slightly different types of support. Under certain conditions each source can provide substitutable support. On the basis of her earlier work on blacks, whites, and Hispanics in New York, Marjorie Cantor (1979) drew similar conclusions. Litwak (1985) has extended the notion of substitution by theorizing that loss of network members results in replacements according to a set of specifiable rules. Gibson and Jackson (in press) have also speculated on the competence of the elderly in locating a variety of different support providers.

Griffith (1985) found in a large sample of adults that although family members dominated the networks of their respondents, the most sought-after support provider was a same-sex friend. Prior research has pointed to the important role that the availability of spouse and children play in keeping older individuals out of institutions (Hanson & Sauer, 1985; Johnson & Catalano, 1981; Longino & Lipman, 1981, 1985).

Life-Course Reciprocity and Exchange

The social support literature has reached two fairly firm points of consensus during the last two decades. The first is that social support has to be construed within an interpersonal social relationship framework (e.g., House et al., 1988; Sarason et al., 1990) and the other is that the roots of such an interpersonal relationship reside in early socialization and attachment processes (e.g., Antonucci, 1990; Sarason et al., 1990). Building on these two points, we (Antonucci, 1985a; Antonucci & Jackson, 1987, 1989, 1990) have speculated on a model of social exchange that takes as its premise the development of rudimentary social relationships as a function of the attachment experience, reinforcement in adolescence, maturity in early to mid-adulthood and adjustment and reorientation with the diminishment of personal resources in later stages of the life-span. Using an exchange and reciprocity model, we argue that individuals "bank" resources gained from interaction with others in earlier points of the life-course and call on these resources in later periods when failing health, disability, and a diminishment of other resources may not permit strict rules of reciprocity to be followed in interpersonal interactions. We believe that this "banking" and later "withdrawal" may be obviously true for tangible resources (aid), but may be more critically important for the more emotionally (affirmation) and feeling (affect)-based dimensions of social supportive behaviors.

Thus, to understand the nature of interpersonal relationships in older age, one must understand the nature of the individual history of transactions with others in the network (George, 1986). This is critical to the extent to which personal accounting systems of tangible, emotional, and affective supports given at earlier periods in the life course permit individuals to take from others freely and without feelings of unequal obligation (indebtedness) in what become unequal and nonreciprocal relationships. We believe that this conceptualization within a developmental schema may account for a wide divergence of findings in the field. These include the apparent volitional diminishment, at times, of the size of the network in older years: the effects of the confidant and qualitative changes in the use of only parts of the network; processes by which some supportive behaviors are perceived as negative; and the maintenance of interpersonal relationships of a nonreciprocal nature in the face of strong societal pressures to maintain equality in personal interactions.

Mechanisms of Social Support Effectiveness

Although some unanimity now exists regarding the framework for construing the social and interpersonal boundaries of the context for socially supportive behavioral exchanges, less agreement exists on how and why social support is effective in the health and well-being of the elderly (Antonucci & Jackson, 1987; Antonucci & Johnson, in press; Coyne & Bolger, 1990). Although we have speculated on possible physiological mechanisms that may play a role in carrying the effects of psychological changes, how these individual psychological changes occur is still at issue (Kiecolt-Glazer et al., 1985). Many have speculated on the role of "perceived" support in contrast to received support as a major factor (e.g., Sarason et al., 1990). Others have suggested that changes in coping resources (Pearlin, 1989; Thoits,

1982, 1984, 1986), and changes in esteem and personal efficacy (e.g., Krause, 1990) may serve as possible mediators of support received.

There seems little doubt that perceived control may play an important role in an individual's assessment of, and adjustment to, the environment (Hamburg, Elliot, & Parron, 1982; Janis & Rodin, 1979; Schaie, Rodin, & Schooler, 1990; Skinner, 1985). Several studies have shown effects of personal efficacy and control on such divergent areas as persistence (Jacobs, Prentice-Dunn, & Rogers, 1984); and engaging in health behaviors (Abella & Heslin, 1984). Some negative evidence, however, suggests that in certain situations excessive perceptions and need for control may lead to poor behavioral choices (Miller, Lack, & Asroff, 1985).

A great deal of research has specifically addressed the issue of control with older people (Baltes, 1982; Baltes & Baltes, 1986; Janis & Rodin, 1979; Lachman, 1985; Schaie et al., 1990). The findings are clear that inducing feelings of autonomy and control in older persons may lead to reduced morbidity and improved chances of survival (e.g., Langer & Rodin, 1976; Schulz, 1976). Several studies have demonstrated a relationship between domain-specific self-efficacy and health (Atkins, Kaplan, Timms, Reinsch, & Lofback, in press; Bandura, 1982; Ewart, Taylor, Reese, & DeBusk, 1983; Kaplan, Atkins, & Reinsch, 1984; O'Leary, 1985).

We have noted earlier (Antonucci & Jackson, 1987) that this body of research is most often considered as an intraindividual psychological process (e.g., Lachman, 1985). We believe, however, that its most important implications are for the interindividual and social psychological processes undergirding the nature of socially supportive behaviors (Lemke & Moos, 1981; Moos, 1981; Moos & Igra, 1980). Several researchers have proposed and tested whether social support might be related to some other stable personality characteristic such as self-esteem, mastery, or personal competence (Antonucci, 1990; Gore, 1985; Heller, 1986; Jung, 1984; Pearlin, 1985; Reis, 1984; Krause, 1990; Wills, 1985). We believe that these research findings are uncontestable in showing that supportive relationships foster, develop, and help maintain in the elderly a perception and sense of control and self. What we believe has been missing in the social support literature is the explicit recognition and incorporation of the social psychological aspects of the social support situation (Antonucci & Jackson, 1987). We have suggested that the social support situation is at least in fact or symbolically one of minimum social interaction. Thus, it involves as a minimum a support recipient and support provider (see Brehm, 1984, for a similar model). Considerations of larger networks are only extensions of this basic situation. The research by Lowenthal and Haven (1968) has suggested that it is the minimal social situation (i.e., confidant relationship) that is most important in the provision of social support. This finding is consistent with the support-efficacy framework that we have proposed in greater detail elsewhere (Antonucci & Jackson, 1987).

Much of the support literature has focused on the nature of the support network (e.g., structure, function, etc.) or on the perceived quantity or quality of support received by the recipient (Sarason et al., 1990). Less work has focused on the relationship between support provider and support recipient in terms of factors that may influence the nature and effectiveness of the support provider's behaviors. Thus, equivalent "supportive behaviors" engaged in by different support providers may be differentially perceived and effective in the support relationship (Antonucci, 1985a; Antonucci & Jackson, 1987). This hypothesized process may account for why equivalent behaviors are differentially effective and even why tangible support may not always result in positive outcomes.

We believe that the willingness of the support provider to engage in what appear to be supportive behaviors is a complex process that begins with the support provider's beliefs about the perceived efficacy of the target person to engage in the relevant behaviors. This perception may be affected by objective indicators in the environment but also may be dependent on the prior relationship between the provider and recipient, and the ability and willingness of the recipient to engage in the behaviors.

Similarly, this approach also takes into consideration perceptual and cognitive factors in the relationship between support provider and support recipient. Thus, it can also explain why some ostensibly supportive behaviors can be construed as negative support (Heller, 1979; Rook, 1985, 1990). In some situations it may be that the attributions of a support recipient regarding the legitimacy of the motivation(s) underlying the behaviors are most important. In short, not all supportive behaviors engaged in by the support provider will be positively evaluated or have positive effects on the personal efficacy of the support recipient. If these positive effects on the personal efficacy of the support recipient do not occur, then the behaviors of the support recipient are not supportive according to our definition of the concept. In fact, negative support can be viewed as not only the absence of influence on the self-efficacy of the support recipient but also as an actual decrease in the self-efficacy of the support recipient.

The proposed framework may also help to account for many disparate findings in the literature—for example, the greater predictive power of adequacy and perception over structural or functional measures of social support, and why quantity of support appears to be less effective, proportionately, than quality of support. As has often been shown in the literature (e.g., Lowenthal & Haven, 1968) quality of perceived support is important, perhaps because the confidant communicates and promotes the recipient's self-efficacy.

We believe the proposed support-efficacy framework can begin to account for some of the seemingly contradictory findings in the social support literature. The conceptualization is consistent with the work that has demonstrated effects of control and efficacy on a wide variety of outcomes, particularly health and health-related behaviors (Atkins et al., in press; Baltes & Baltes, 1986; Ewart et al., 1983; Kaplan et al., 1984; Krause, 1990; Langer & Rodin, 1976; Rodin, 1980; Schaie et al., 1990; Schulz, 1976; Thomas, Garry, Goodwin, & Goodwin, 1985). We believe that measures based on the proposed support-efficacy framework will be more useful in accounting for health and other successful outcomes in elderly populations than traditional structure and function measures of social support.

The support-efficacy model is also compatible with the life-course reciprocity, support-bank framework described earlier. Lifetime patterns of social interaction and perceptions of appropriateness and motivations for exchanges, we believe, play themselves out in the type of intense psychological and cognitive model we have described (Antonucci & Jackson, 1987). It is this psychological process that may ultimately result in both psychological and physiological changes that affect the future course of both health and effective functioning.

CONCLUSION

In this chapter we attempted a critical review of the social support literature as it related to health and effective functioning in the elderly. There seems to be little doubt that socially supportive processes, both in the face of stressful events and in their absence, play significant roles in the health and well-being of the elderly. We suggested that the structure, function, reciprocal relationships, source of support, actual versus perceived support, veridicality of perception of support, and network enmeshment all play critical roles in understanding the nature of supportive exchanges in older age. We attempted to explore the role that different sources of support may play both in buffering these stressors and as a source of generalized, positive emotional succorance, as well as possible mechanisms through which socially supportive behaviors and their receipt may have their beneficial and negative effects. We noted the lack of attention of previous research to both social support as a dependent variable (a point noted especially in Krause & Keith, 1989) and in its effects on health and well-being of the elderly.

We noted confusion in the definition and measurement of social support and highlighted recent attempts to define and measure the construct in a multidimensional manner (e.g., Dean et al., 1989). We also suggested that although there have been some longitudinal studies of social support (Antonucci, 1991), the lack of consistent measurement and long-term observations of change make an evaluative assessment of these data still problematic. We believe, however, that it can be concluded that both continuity and change (Field & Minkler, 1988) probably characterize the nature of interpersonal and supportive relationships in older ages, and that a combination of availability of resources (Morgan, 1988), substitutability of helpers (Cantor, 1979; Gibson & Jackson, in press; Taylor, 1985), and the nature of interpersonal and supportive relationships during the life course (Antonucci, 1990) all play an important role in understanding the nature, and contributing to the appropriate measurement, of social support in older ages.

The social support process is of critical practical concern in the delivery of services to the elderly and to an increasingly older population of potentially frail individuals. An ever-growing impoverished society will find it difficult to continue to increase resources to care for this population. Conversely, data clearly show both a preference for and strong sources of informal support for the elderly (Stephens et al., 1990). Changes in family composition, increased level of burdens, reduced resources in younger members of intergenerational networks, especially among some racial and ethnic population groups (Jackson et al., 1990), however, lead to the inescapable conclusion that ways of increasing the effectiveness of the available support from both informal and formal sources must be found.

We suggest that future research should focus on the mechanisms that undergird the sources and nature of supportive behaviors, intra-personal and interpersonal dynamics of social support exchange processes, and the social and psychological processes that may hinder or promote the effectiveness of ostensibly socially supportive behaviors in the health and effective functioning of the elderly.

We believe that processes of social support have to be conceptualized and researched within a life-span or life-course theoretical framework. We suggested that history of personal interactions, nature of prior support networks, and the nature of exchanges, like the support bank, demand a much more dynamic life-course treatment than is currently provided by most theorists. Within this conception we then highlighted the importance of reciprocity relationships, the need to distinguish clearly quality from quantity of support and structural from functional relationships. Perhaps most important is the need to begin the difficult process of addressing the nature of the mechanism(s) through which social relationships and socially supportive behaviors have their effects on health and effective functioning among the elderly.

REFERENCES

Abella, R., & Heslin, R. (1984). Health, locus of control, values, and the behavior of family and friends: An integrated approach to understanding preventive health behavior. *Basic and Applied Social Psychology, 5,* 283–293.

Ader, R., & Cohen, N. (1984). Behavior and the immune system. In W. D. Gentry (Ed.), *Handbook of behavioral medicine* (pp. 117–173). New York: Guilford Press.

Antonucci, T. C. (1985a). Personal characteristics, social support, and social behavior. In R. H. Binstock & E. Shanas (Eds.), *Handbook of aging and the social sciences* (2nd ed., pp. 94–128). New York: Van Nostrand Reinhold.

Antonucci, T. C. (1985b). Social support: Theoretical advances, recent findings and pressing issues. In I. G. Sarason & B. R. Sarason (Eds.), *Social support: Theory, research, and applications* (pp. 21–57). Dordrecht, The Netherlands: Martinus Nijhoff.

Antonucci, T. C. (1989). Social support and the disease process. In L. L. Carstensen & J. M. Neale (Eds.), *Mechanisms of psychological influence on physical health: With special attention to the elderly* (pp. 23–41). New York: Plenum.

Antonucci, T. C. (1990). Social supports and social relationships. In R. H. Binstock & L. K. George (Eds.), *Handbook of aging and the social sciences* (3rd ed., pp. 205–227). New York: Academic Press.

Antonucci, T. C. (1991). Attachment, social support and coping with negative life events in mature adulthood. In E. M. Cummings, A. L. Greene, & K. H. Karraker (Eds.), *Life-span developmental psychology: Vol. 11. Stress and coping across the life-span* (pp. 261–275). Hillsdale, NJ: Erlbaum.

Antonucci, T. C., & Depner, C. E. (1982). Social support and informal helping relationships. In T. A. Wills (Ed.), *Basic processes in helping relationships* (pp. 233–254). New York: Academic Press.

Antonucci, T. C., & Jackson, J. S. (1987). Social support, interpersonal efficacy, and health: A life course perspective. In L. L. Carstensen & B. A. Edelstein (Eds.), *Handbook of clinical gerontology* (pp. 292–311). New York: Pergamon.

Antonucci, T. C., & Jackson, J. S. (1989). Successful ageing and life course reciprocity. In A. W. Warnes (Ed.), *Human ageing and later life: Multidisciplinary perspectives* (pp. 83–95). London: Edward Arnold, a Division of Hodder & Soughton Educational.

Antonucci, T. C., & Jackson, J. S. (1990). The role of reciprocity in social support. In B. R. Sarason, I. G. Sarason, & G. R. Pierce (Eds.), *Social support: An interactional view* (pp. 173–198). New York: Wiley & Sons.

Antonucci, T. C., & Johnson, E. H. (in press). Conceptualization and methods in social support theory and research as related to cardiovascular disease. In S. A. Schumaker & S. M. Czajkowski (Eds.), *Social support and cardiovascular disease*. New York: Plenum Press.

Atkins, C., Kaplan, R. M., Timms, R. M., Reinsch, S., & Lofback, K. (in press). Behavioral programs for exercise compliance in chronic obstructive pulmonary disease. *Journal of Consulting and Clinical Psychology*.

Baltes, M. M. (1982). Environmental factors in dependency among nursing home residents: A social ecology analysis. In T. A. Wills (Ed.), *Basic processes in helping relationships* (pp. 405–425). New York: Academic Press.

Baltes, M. M., & Baltes, P. B. (Eds.). (1986). *The psychology of control and aging*. Hillsdale, NJ: Erlbaum.

Bandura, A. (1982). Self-efficacy mechanism in human agency. *American Psychologist, 37*, 122–147.

Berkman, L. F. (1984). Assessing the physical health effects of social networks and social support. *Annual Review of Public Health, 5*, 413–432.

Berkman, L. F., & Syme, S. L. (1979). Social networks, host resistance, and mortality: A nine-year follow-up study of Alameda County residents. *American Journal of Epidemiology, 109*, 186–204.

Biegel, D. E. (1985). The application of network theory and research to the field of aging. In W. J. Sauer & R. T. Coward (Eds.), *Social support networks and the care of the elderly* (pp. 251–273). New York: Springer.

Blazer, D. G. (1982). Social support and mortality in an elderly population. *American Journal of Epidemiology, 115,* 684–694.

Boissevain, J. (1974). *Friends of friends: Networks, manipulators and coalitions.* New York: St. Martin's Press.

Bott, E. (1957). *Family and social network: Roles, norms and external relationships in ordinary urban families.* London: Tavistock Institute of Human Relations.

Brehm, S. S. (1984). Social support processes. In J. C. Masters & K. Yarkin-Levin (Eds.), *Boundary areas in social and developmental psychology* (pp. 107–129). New York: Academic Press.

Brownell, A., & Shumaker, S. A. (1984). Social support: An introduction to a complex phenomenon. *Journal of Social Issues, 40,* 1–10.

Brubaker, T. H. (1990). A contextual approach to the development of stress associated with care-giving in later-life families (pp. 29–47). In M. A. P. Stephens, J. H. Crowther, S. E. Hobfoll, & D. L. Tennenbaum (Eds.), *Stress and coping in later-life families.* New York: Hemisphere.

Cantor, M. H. (1979). Neighbors and friends: An overlooked resource in the informal support system. *Research on Aging, 1,* 434–463.

Cassel, J. (1976). The contribution of the social environment to host resistance. *American Journal of Epidemiology, 104,* 107–123.

Chappell, N. L. (1983). Informal support networks among the elderly. *Research on Aging, 5,* 77–99.

Cobb, S. (1976). Social support as a moderator of life stress. *Psychsomatic Medicine, 38,* 300–314.

Cohen, C. I., & Rajkowski, H. (1982). What's in a friend? Substantive and theoretical issues. *The Gerontologist, 22,* 261–266.

Cohen, S., & Wills, T. A. (1985). Stress, social support, and the buffering hypothesis. *Psychological Bulletin, 98,* 310–357.

Coyne, J. C., & Bolger, N. (1990). Doing without social support as an explanatory concept. *Journal of Social and Clinical Psychology, 9,* 148–158.

Coyne, J. C., & DeLongis, A. (1986). Going beyond social support: The role of social relationships in adaptation. *Journal of Consulting and Clinical Psychology, 54,* 454–460.

Coyne, J. C., & Downey, G. (1991). Social factors and psychopathology: Stress, social support, and coping processes. *Annual Review of Psychology, 42,* 401–425.

Coyne, J. C., Ellard, J. H., & Smith, D. A. F. (1990). Social support, interdependence, and the dilemmas of helping. In B. R. Sarason, I. G. Sarason, & G. R. Pierce (Eds.), *Social support: An interactional view* (pp. 129–149). New York: Wiley & Sons.

Coyne, J. C., & Gotlib, I. H. (1983). The role of cognition in depression: A critical appraisal. *Psychological Bulletiln, 94,* 472–505.

Crohan, S. E., & Antonucci, T. C. (1989). Friends as a source of social support in old age. In R. G. Adams & R. Blieszner (Eds.), *Older adult friendship* (pp. 129–146). Beverly Hills: Sage.

D'Augelli, A. (1983). Social support networks in mental health. In J. K. Whittaker, J. Garbarino, & Associates (Eds.), *Social support networks: Informal helping in the human services* (pp. 71–106). New York: Aldine.

Dean, A., Kolody, B., Wood, P., & Ensel, W. M. (1989). Measuring the communication of social support from adult children. *Journal of Gerontology, Social Sciences, 44,* S71–79.

Depner, C. E., Wethington, E., & Ingersoll-Dayton, B. (1984). Social support: Methodological issues in design and measurement. *Journal of Social Issues, 40,* 37–54.

Duff, R. W., & Hong, L. K. (1982). Quality and quantity of social interactions in the life satisfaction of older Americans. *Sociology and Social Research, 66,* 418–434.

Ewart, C. K., Taylor, C. B., Reese, L. B., & DeBusk, R. F. (1983). Effects of early postmyocardial infarction exercise testing on self-perception and subsequent physical activity. *American Journal of Cardiology, 51,* 1076–1080.

Felton, B., Lehmann, S., Adler, A., & Burgio, M. (1981). Single room occupancy hotels: Their viability as housing options for older citizens. In M. P. Lawton & S. L. Hoover (Eds.), *Community housing choices for older Americans* (pp. 267–285). New York: Springer.

Ferraro, K. F., Mutran, E., & Barresi, C. M. (1984). Widowhood, health, and friendship support in later life. *Journal of Health and Social Behavior, 25,* 245–259.

Field, D., & Minkler, M. (1988). Continuity and change in social support between young-old and old-old or very-old age. *Journal of Gerontology: Psychological Sciences, 43,* P100–106.

French, J. R. P., Jr. (1974). Person-role fit. In A. McLean (Ed.), *Occupational stress* (pp. 70–79). Springfield, IL: Charles C Thomas.

George, L. K. (1986). Caregiver burden: Conflict between norms of reciprocity and solidarity. In K. A. Pillemer & R. S. Wolf (Eds.), *Elder abuse: Conflict in the family* (pp. 67–92). Dover, MA: Auburn House.

Gibson, R. C., & Jackson, J. S. (in press). The black oldest old: Informal support, physical, psychological, and social functioning. In R. Suzman, D. Willis, & K. Manton (Eds.), *The oldest old.* New York: Oxford Press.

Gore, L. (1985). Social support and styles of coping with stress. In S. Cohen & S. L. Syme (Eds.), *Social support and health* (pp. 263–278). New York: Academic Press.

Gottlieb, B. H. (1981). *Social networks and social support.* Beverly Hills, CA: Sage.

Greenblatt, M., Becerra, R. M., & Serafetinides, E. A. (1982). Social networks and mental health: An overview. *American Journal of Psychiatry, 139,* 977-984.

Griffith, J. (1985). Social support providers: Who are they? Where are they met? And the relationship of network characteristics to psychological distress. *Basic and Applied Social Psychology, 6,* 41-60.

Hamburg, D. A., Elliot, G. R., & Parron, D. L. *Health and behavior: Frontiers of research in the biobehavioral sciences.* Washington, DC: National Academy Press.

Hanson, S. H., & Sauer, W. G. (1985). Children and their elderly parents. In W. J. Sauer & R. T. Coward (Eds.), *Social support networks and the care of the elderly* (pp. 41-66). New York: Springer.

Haug, M. R., Breslau, N., & Folmar, S. J. (1989). Coping resources and selective survival in mental health of the elderly. *Research on Aging, 11,* 468-491.

Heller, K. (1979). The effects of social support: Prevention and treatment implications. In A. P. Goldstein & F. H. Kanfer (Eds.), *Maximizing treatment gains: Transfer enhancement in psychotherapy* (pp. 353-382). New York: Academic Press.

Heller, K. (1986). Introduction to the special series. *Journal of Consulting and Clinical Psychology, 54,* 415.

Heller, K., & Mansbach, W. E. (1984). The multifaceted nature of social support in a community sample of elderly women. *Journal of Social Issues, 40,* 99-112.

Hobfoll, S. E., & Freedy, J. R. (1990). The availability and effective use of social support. *Journal of Social and Clinical Psychology, 9,* 91-103.

House, J. S., & Kahn, R. L. (1985). Measures and concepts of social support. In S. Cohen & S. L. Syme (Eds.), *Social support and health* (pp. 83-108). New York: Academic Press.

House, J. S., Robbins, C., & Metzner, H. L. (1982). The association of social relationships and activities with mortality: Prospective evidence from the Tecumseh Community Health Study. *American Journal of Epidemiology, 116,* 123-140.

House, J. S., Umberson, D., & Landis, K. R. (1988). Structures and processes of social support. *Annual Review of Sociology, 14,* 293-318.

Huber, J., & Spitze, G. (1988). Trends in family sociology. In N. J. Smelser (Ed.), *Handbook of sociology* (pp. 425-448). Beverly Hills: Sage.

Ishii-Kuntz, M., & Seccombe, K. (1989). The impact of children upon social support networks throughout the life course. *Journal of Marriage and the Family, 51,* 777-790.

Jackson, J. S. (Ed.). (1988). *The black American elderly: Research on physical and psychosocial health.* New York: Springer.

Jackson, J. S., Antonucci, T. C., & Gibson, R. C. (1990). Cultural, racial, and ethnic minority influences on aging. In J. E. Birren & K. W. Schaie (Eds.), *Handbook of the psychology of aging* (3rd ed., pp. 103–123). New York: Academic Press.

Jacobs, B., Prentice-Dunn, S., & Rogers, R. W. (1984). Understanding persistence: An interface of control theory and self-efficacy theory. *Basic and Applied Social Psychology, 5,* 333–347.

Janis, I. L., & Rodin, J. (1979). Attribution, control, and decision making: Social psychology and health care. In G. C. Stone, S. M. Weiss, J. D. Matarazzo, N. E. Miller, J. Rodin, C. D. Belar, M. J. Follick, & J. E. Singer (Eds.), *Health psychology: A handbook* (pp. 487–521). San Francisco: Jossey-Bass Publishers.

Jemmott, J., & Locke, S. E. (1984). Psychosocial factors, immunologic mediation, and human susceptibility to infectious diseases: How much do we know? *Psychological Bulletin, 95,* 78–108.

Johnson, C. L., & Catalano, D. J. (1981). Childless elderly and their family supports. *The Gerontologist, 21,* 610–618.

Jones, B. (1981). *Mental health and the structure of support.* Unpublished doctoral dissertation, The University of Michigan, Ann Arbor.

Jung, J. (1984). Social support and its relation to health: A critical evaluation. *Basic and Applied Social Psychology, 5,* 143–169.

Kaplan, R. M., Atkins, C. J., & Reinsch, S. (1984). Specific efficacy expectations mediate exercise compliance in patients with COPD. *Health Psychology, 3,* 223–242.

Kasl, S. V., & Berkman, L. F. (1981). Some psychosocial influences on the health status of the elderly: The perspective of social epidemiology. In J. L. McCaugh & S. B. Kiesler (Eds.), *Aging: Biology and behavior* (pp. 345–385). New York: Academic Press.

Kessler, R. C., Price, R. H., & Wortman, C. B. (1985). Social factors in psychopathology: Stress, social support, and coping processes. *Annual Review of Psychology, 36,* 531–572.

Kiecolt-Glaser, J. K., Glaser, R., Williger, D., Stout, J., Messick, G., Sheppard, S., Ricker, D., Romisher, S. C., Briner, W., Bonnell, G., & Donnerberg, R. (1985). Psychosocial enhancement of immunocompetence in a geriatric population. *Health Psychology, 4,* 25–41.

Kiesler, C. A. (1985). Policy implications of research on social support and health. In S. Cohen & S. L. Syme (Eds.), *Social support and health* (pp. 347–364). New York: Academic Press.

Krause, N. (1990). Stress, support, and well-being in later life: Focusing on salient social roles. In M. A. P. Stephens, J. H. Crowther, S. E. Hobfoll, & D. L. Tennenbaum (Eds.), *Stress and coping in later-life families* (pp. 71–97). New York: Hemisphere.

Krause, N., & Keith, V. (1989). Gender differences in social support among older adults. *Sex Roles, 21,* 609–628.

Kreppner, K. (1989). Linking infant development-in-context research to the investigation of life-span family development. In K. Kreppner & R. M. Lerner (Eds.), *Family systems and life-span development* (pp. 33–64). Hillsdale, NJ: Erlbaum.

Lachman, M. E. (1985). Personal efficacy in middle and old age: Differential and normative patterns of change. In G. H. Elder, Jr. (Ed.), *Life course dynamics* (pp. 188–213). Ithaca, NY: Cornell University Press.

Langer, E. J., & Rodin, J. (1976). The effects of choice and enhanced personal responsibility for the aged: A field experiment in an institutional setting. *Journal of Personality and Social Psychology, 34,* 191–198.

Lee, G. R., & Shehan, C. L. (1989). Social relations and the self-esteem of older persons. *Research on Aging, 11,* 427–442.

Lemke, S., & Moos, R. H. (1981). The suprapersonal environments of sheltered care settings. *Journal of Gerontology, 26,* 233–243.

Levitt, M. J., Antonucci, T. C., Clark, M. C., Rotton, J., & Finley, G. E. (1985). Social support and well-being: Preliminary indicators based on two samples of the elderly. *International Journal of Aging and Human Development, 21,* 61–77.

Litwak, E. (1985). *Helping the elderly: The complementary roles of informal networks and formal systems.* New York: Guilford Press.

Longino, C. F., Jr., & Lipman, A. (1981). Married and spouseless men and women in planned retirement communities: Support network differentials. *Journal of Marriage and the Family, 43,* 169–177.

Longino, C. F., Jr., & Lipman, A. (1985). The support systems of women. In W. J. Sauer & R. T. Coward (Eds.), *Social support networks and the care of the elderly* (pp. 219–233). New York: Springer.

Lowenthal, M. F., & Haven, C. (1968). Interaction and adaptation: Intimacy as a critical variable. *American Sociological Review, 33,* 20–30.

Lubben, J. E., & Becerra, R. M. (1987). Social support among black, Mexican, and Chinese elderly. In D. E. Gelfand & C. M. Barresi (Eds.), *Ethnic dimensions of aging* (pp. 130–144). New York: Springer.

McFarlane, A. H., Norman, G. R., Streiner, D. L., & Roy, R. G. (1984). Characteristics and correlates of effective and ineffective social supports. *Journal of Psychosomatic Research, 28,* 501–510.

Mermelstein, B., Cohen, S., & Lichtenstein, E., Baer, J. S., & Kamarck, T. (1986). Social support and smoking cessation and maintenance. *Journal of Consulting and Clinical Psychology, 54,* 447–453.

Miller, S. M., Lack, E. R., & Asroff, S. (1985). Preference for control and the coronary-prone behavior pattern: "I'd rather do it myself." *Journal of Psychiatry and Social Psychology, 49,* 492–499.

Moos, R. H. (1981). Environment choice and control in community care settings for older people. *Journal of Applied Psychology, 11,* 23–43.

Moos, R., & Igra, A. (1980). Determinants of the social environments of sheltered care settings. *Journal of Health and Social Behavior, 21,* 88–98.

Morgan, D. L. (1988). Age differences in social network participation. *Journal of Gerontology: Social Sciences, 43,* S129–137.

O'Leary, A. (1985). Self-efficacy and health. *Behavior Research and Therapy, 23,* 437–451.

Pearlin, L. I. (1985). Social structure and processes of social support. In S. Cohen & S. L. Syme (Eds.), *Social support and health* (pp. 43–60). New York: Academic Press.

Pearlin, L. I. (1989). The sociological study of stress. *Journal of Health and Social Behavior, 30,* 241–256.

Pearlin, L. I., Mullan, J. T., Semple, S. J., & Skaff, M. M. (1990). Caregiving and the stress process: An overview of concepts and their measures. *The Gerontologist, 30,* 583–594.

Porritt, D. (1979). Social support in crises: Quantity or quality. *Social Science and Medicine, 13*(A), 715–721.

Rathbone-McCuan, E. E., Hooyman, N., & Fortune, A. E. (1985). Social support for the frail elderly. In W. J. Sauer & R. T. Coward (Eds.), *Social support networks and the care of the elderly* (pp. 234–247). New York: Springer.

Reis, H. T. (1984). Social interaction and well-being. In S. W. Duck (Ed.), *Personal relationships: Repairing personal relationships* (pp. 21–45). New York: Academic Press.

Revicki, D. A., & Mitchell, J. P. (1990). Strain, social support, and mental health in rural elderly individuals. *Journal of Gerontology: Social Sciences, 45,* S267–274.

Rodin, J. (1980). Managing the stress of aging: The role of control and coping. In S. Levine & H. Ursin (Eds.), *Coping and health* (pp. 171–202). New York: Plenum.

Rook, K. (1985). Research on social support, loneliness, and social isolation: Toward an integration. In P. Shaver (Ed.), *Review of personality and social psychology: Emotions, relationships and health* (Vol. 5, pp. 239–264). Beverly Hills: Sage.

Rook, K. (1990). Social relationships as a source of companionship: Implications for older adults' psychological well-being. In B. R. Sarason, I. G. Sarason, & G. R. Pierce (Eds.), *Social support: An interactional view* (pp. 219–250). New York: Wiley & Sons.

Sarason, B. R., Sarason, I. G., & Pierce, G. R. (1990). Traditional views of social support and their impact on assessment. In B. R. Sarason, I. G. Sarason, & G. R. Pierce (Eds.), *Social support: An interactional view* (pp. 9–25). New York: Wiley & Sons.

Sarason, I. G., & Sarason, B. R. (Eds.). (1985). *Social support: Theory, research and applications.* Dordrecht, The Netherlands: Martinus Nijhoff.

Schaie, K. W., Rodin, J., & Schooler, C. (1990). *Self-directedness: Cause and effects throughout the life course.* Hillsdale, NJ: Erlbaum.

Schulz, R. (1976). Effects of control and predictability on the physical and psychological well-being of the institutionalized aged. *Journal of Personality and Social Psychology, 33,* 563–573.

Seeman, T. E., & Berkman, L. F. (1988). Structural characteristics of social networks and their relationship with social support in the elderly: Who provides support. *Social Science and Medicine, 26,* 737–749.

Skinner, E. A. (1985). Action, control judgments, and the structure of control experience. *Psychological Review, 92,* 39–58.

Soldo, B. J., & Manton, K. G. (1985). Health status and service needs of the oldest old: Current patterns and future trends. *Milbank Memorial Fund Quarterly, 63,* 286–323.

Stephens, M. A. P., Crowther, J. H., Hobfoll, S. E., & Tennenbaum, D. L. (Eds.). (1990). *Stress and coping in later-life families.* New York: Hemisphere.

Strain, L. A., & Chappell, N. A. (1982). Confidants: Do they make a difference in quality of life? *Research on Aging, 4,* 479–502.

Taylor, R. J. (1985). The extended family as a source of support to elderly blacks. *The Gerontologist, 25,* 488–495.

Thoits, P. A. (1982). Conceptual, methodological and theoretical problems in studying social support as a buffer against life stress. *Journal of Health and Social Behavior, 23,* 145–159.

Thoits, P. A. (1984). Coping, social support, and psychological outcomes: The central role of emotions. In P. Shaver (Ed.), *Review of personality and social psychology: Emotions, relationships, and health* (Vol. 5, pp. 219–238). Beverly Hills: Sage.

Thoits, P. A. (1986). Social support as coping assistance. *Journal of Consulting and Clinical Psychology, 54,* 416–423.

Thomas, P. D., Garry, P. J., Goodwin, J. M., & Goodwin, J. S. (1985). Social bonds in a healthy elderly sample: Characteristics and associated variables. *Social Science and Medicine, 20,* 365–369.

Wan, T. T. H., & Weissert, W. G. (1981). Social support networks, patient status, and institutionalization. *Research on Aging, 3,* 240–256.

Ward, R. A., Sherman, S. R., & LaGory, M. (1984). Informal networks and knowledge of services for older persons. *Journal of Gerontology, 39,* 216–223.

Wills, T. A. (1985). Supportive functions of interpersonal relationships. In S. Cohen & S. L. Syme (Eds.), *Social support and health* (pp. 61–82). New York: Academic Press.

4

Aging, Coping, and Efficacy: Theoretical Framework for Examining Coping in Life-Span Developmental Context

Carolyn M. Aldwin

In the past decade, there has been an increasing interest in the effect of aging on stress and coping processes. As with any such endeavor, the initial steps have involved documenting the existence of differences—do older adults have different experiences of stress than do younger adults, and are there any characteristic differences in the way in which they cope with stress? Several studies have addressed these issues, generally examining cohort differences in stress and coping. As yet, there have been few attempts to place work on stress and coping in a life-span *developmental* context. This chapter represents such an attempt. First, the existing literature on age differences in stress and coping processes is reviewed. Second, the relevance of certain constructs from life-span developmental psychology is applied to the stress and coping literature to provide a theoretical framework for delineating the ways in which adaptation changes during the life-span. Third, hypotheses concerning the ways in which aging can affect the stress and coping process are discussed. Finally, preliminary data from two studies are presented in support of the hypotheses generated from this theoretical framework.

DOES AGE AFFECT THE STRESS PROCESS?

There is little doubt that the nature of stressful experiences changes during the life-span. Older adults are much more likely to experience health declines, with both their own health and that of their family members, and are more likely to be bereaved. They are more likely to exit work roles and less likely to begin new jobs, schooling, or families. There is also some speculation that adults may become less egocentric in the nature of the concerns they report—that is, some adults become more concerned with the problem of loved ones, in keeping with Erikson's construct of generativity (Erikson, 1950; Erikson, Erikson, & Kivnick, 1986). (For reviews of stress and aging, see Aldwin, 1990; Paykel, 1983).

Whether or not age affects the appraisal of stress, however, is a matter of some debate. The elderly are widely assumed to be more external in their control expectancies than are younger adults (c.f., Rodin, 1986), which suggests that they may be likely to appraise stressful situations differently. To the extent that they are more external, they should be less likely to feel in control of situations, and thus more likely to perceive events as threatening or changeable. Accordingly, they should perceive threats as more stressful and their coping efforts as less efficacious.

The support for this hypothesis is, at best, mixed. One early study found that older adults tended to rate life events as being more stressful than do younger adults and suggested that older individuals are more vulnerable to environmental change (Muhlenkamp, Gress, & Flood, 1975). A more recent study using data from the National Health Interview Study found, however, that elderly respondents were less likely than younger ones to report either experiencing stress or that stress had "a lot" of effect on their health (Silverman, Eichler, & Williams, 1987; see also Sands & Parker, 1980).

Lachman (1986) argued that older adults do not differ in general expectancies of control, but rather differ on specific dimensions, such as chance and powerful others. The stress and coping literature appears to support this observation. For example, Blanchard-Fields and Robinson (1987) found no age differences in generalized locus of control, but did find differences with the domains of interpersonal relationships and achievement. In particular, the elderly were less likely to self-attribute controllability for the causes or outcomes of stressful events in these domains. Similarly, Folkman, Lazarus, Pimley, and Novacek (1987) showed that the elderly were less likely to appraise their stressful encounters as changeable than were younger groups.

McCrae (1982) also found age differences in appraisals of stress. However, he cautioned that appraisals of controllability are in part a function of environmental characteristics. Thus, the differences in appraisals seen between older and younger adults may be more of a function of differences in the types of stressors that these groups were facing than any developmental shifts in appraisal processes.

DOES AGE AFFECT THE COPING PROCESS?

Early studies focused on trying to determine whether there were decrements or increments in coping strategies with age. Using Thematic Apperception Tests (TATs) in samples from different cultures, Gutmann (1974) examined developmental shifts in mastery styles. He argued that young adults demonstrated "active" mastery styles, middle-aged adults adopted "passive" mastery styles, and old adults exhibited "magical" mastery styles—that is, their solutions toward problems showed little realism in relation to environmental demands. He found similar trends in several different cultures.

Gutmann's approach is interesting in that he attempted to examine developmental differences in mastery styles cross-culturally, a strategy that is usually reserved for studies of adolescence and only rarely attempted in aging studies. Nonetheless, there are several limitations to interpreting this study as supporting age-related changes in coping strategies. First, it is not clear whether mastery styles identified via TAT responses bear any relationship to actual coping strategies used in stressful situations. For example, generalized expectancies of control generally bear little relationship to control attributions or coping behaviors in actual stressful situations (Folkman, Aldwin, & Lazarus, 1981; Gatz, Siegler, George, & Tyler, 1986).

Second, contrasting cohort differences of mastery styles cross-culturally may be confounded with cultural change, in that older cohorts may be more traditional in their beliefs and values, and younger cohorts more modern (e.g., Inkeles & Smith, 1974). For example, in some non-Western cultures, there is a preference for indirect as opposed to direct action. Rather than using confrontational tactics with interpersonal problems, individuals in Asian cultures may prefer to use intermediaries or other indirect manipulations (Reynolds, 1976). Both direct and indirect action are active problem-solving techniques; they merely differ in the preferred locus of action (c.f., Aldwin, 1986). Gutmann may have confused the preference for indirect action with "passive" or "magical" mastery; the trend for younger adults in Gutmann's non-Western samples for "active" mastery may have simply reflected the greater familiarity of the young to Western culture. Thus, cultural change may have been mistaken for developmental change.

Conversely, it is also possible that the phenomenon that Gutmann observed may truly reflect a developmental shift in coping strategies, not from active to "magical" mastery styles but rather from preferences for direct to indirect action. Whether this actually occurs, and if it would be considered a decrement or increment in coping ability with age, is a matter of debate.

Vaillant (1977) suggested that there were incremental shifts in coping strategies with age. He examined longitudinal changes in the Grant Study men, rating open-ended interview material for the presence of different types of defense mechanisms. The defensive strategies used by younger adults were often deemed "immature" or "neurotic," in that they were more likely to distort reality. By middle age, most men had shifted toward "mature" defensive styles, characterized by less distortion of reality and greater use of positive mechanisms such as sublimation and humor.

Vaillant's study is extremely valuable in that it is the only long-term longitudinal study of coping strategies. Nonetheless, there are certain limitations to this work. The sample is very selective; only white men at a prestigious institution were included, and only selected materials were rated. Further, interrater reliabilities for certain defense mechanisms, especially denial, were very low. Defense mechanisms are only one aspect of adaptive behavior—age changes in problem-focused coping were not addressed. Nonetheless, there is a certain intuitive appeal to the hypothesis that as people mature, their stances toward problems also mature.

Much of the most recent work in the aging and coping literature has focused on actual strategies used by adults in handling problems that occur in their everyday lives. Most studies have shown that there are very few age differences in coping strategies and, for the most part, have concluded that older adults are just as effective copers as younger adults (e.g., Aldwin & Revenson, 1985; Felton & Revenson,

1987; Folkman et al., 1987; Irion & Blanchard-Fields, 1987; McCrae, 1982).

In the absence of any general theory of how stress appraisals and coping strategies change over the life-span, however, we have yet to develop age-sensitive instruments. Thus, there may be developmental changes in appraisal and coping processes that we have not as yet observed.

STRESS AND COPING
IN DEVELOPMENTAL CONTEXT

As Baltes (1987) pointed out, one of the central conundrums for a theory of life-span development is whether or not development actually occurs in adulthood. On the one hand, sociologists such as Featherman and Lerner (1985) argue that there is no universal developmental sequence in adulthood, as cultures and roles within a culture vary so widely that there is no general sequence of stages that adults go through. Conversely, psychologists such as White (1974), Loevinger (1977), and Erikson (1950) described a phenomenon that they believed to be universal. Although they used different terms— mastery, ego development or integrity, and wisdom—and often had different assumptions about the nature of this phenomenon, they all proposed a developmental process that occurred primarily in adulthood. So, the question becomes, how can there be universal developmental processes in adulthood when the context for that development varies so widely across cultures?[1]

Henry and Neugarten (1955) once observed that if one truly wanted to understand a person's personality, then one should examine that person under stress. That observation has led me to examine more closely the role of stress and coping in personality development over the life-span, which has generated several hypotheses.

---

[1]Although cultures also vary for children, the developmental tasks tend to be more universal, such as language acquisition, cognitive development, and the nurturing of social ties. What constitutes the "ideal" adult, however, varies greatly across cultures (c.f., Erikson, 1978), and between social roles within a culture (c.f., Wallace, 1970). Thus, it becomes much more difficult to specify universal tasks in adulthood that are primarily psychological in nature.

First, stressful experiences provide a universal *context* in which adult development can occur. As is commonly observed, stress is ubiquitous and universal (e.g., Selye, 1956). People in all cultures and in all walks of society experience stress—whether that stress derives from frustrated goals, bereavement, conflict with family and friends, loss of self-esteem, economic hardship, or illness. The *content* of a stressful experience or how it is appraised may vary across cultures, but the *experience* itself is universal. A normal consequence of living in any culture is the experience of stress, and it would be difficult to conceive of a role within a culture which is stress free. Thus, stressful experiences warrant closer examination for their developmental implications.

Second, the process of coping with stress may provide a *means* through which development can occur in adulthood. That is, as people cope with stress, they *can*—although they do not necessarily—develop capacities and skills that are prized by a given culture, what Baltes (1987) termed "practical knowledge." This does not mean that there is a "right" way of coping with stress that is developed across the life-span. As Pearlin and Schooler (1978) pointed out, it is unlikely that we will discover a "magic bullet" that could be considered efficacious coping across situations. It is even less likely that there would be a "magic bullet" that would always be appropriate across cultures. Rather, through coping with problems, people can develop "practical knowledge" concerning ways of handling the types of problems that are likely to come up in a given culture, in a manner that is appropriate to that culture.

Third, there is no universal sequence of adult development because, to a large extent, whether development occurs in adulthood is largely a matter of *volition* (c.f., Brandtstädter, Krampen, & Heil, 1986). Not everyone develops wisdom or practical knowledge. How we cope with problems is, to a certain extent, a matter of choice. We can refuse to expend the effort required for an optimal solution, or we can use strategies that maximize our own goals but that involve certain costs, such as the alienation of others. We can deny or refuse to deal with a particular problem by removing ourselves from the context or by shifting the problem to others, such as co-workers, spouses, or siblings. In desperate cases, we may retreat into insanity (c.f., Haan, 1978). By doing so, however, we deprive ourselves of the opportunity to learn, if only from our own mistakes, and to develop skills such as empathy, patience, and courage. These skills, in turn, can be used as resources in coping with future problems.[2] In short, the choices that we make in stressful situations affect future efficacy expectations and adaptive processes.

Thus, by taking a developmental approach to the stress and coping process, the potentially positive aspects of stress can be considered. The idea of positive changes resulting from stressful experiences is not at all new (Moos & Schaefer, 1986). Both Aldwin and Stokols (1988) and Dienstbier (1989) have recently reviewed the relevant clinical and experimental literature concerning positive consequences of exposure to stress. Further, this theme is often expressed in the popular literature, folk wisdom, fairy tales, and even 19th-century novels, to name but a few instances. For example, in Hawthorne's *House of Seven Gables*, the author declares that the heroine's true beauty only emerges after sorrow and grief have tempered and ennobled her spirit.

Both Lieberman (chapter 6) and Kahana (chapter 7) in this book have observed positive changes emerging from the older adults they studied. Lieberman examined the process of adapting to widowhood among older women. He observed that many of the women exhibited gains or growth as a result of this traumatic experience. These included expanding social networks, returning to school, or starting new careers. Kahana, in a study of the long-term effects of the Holocaust, observed that many of these older men had more stable marriages, closer family ties, and more successful careers than individuals who had not undergone the Holocaust. Although this may reflect survivor effects, these results are similar to those found by Elder (1974) in a study of children of the 1930s depression. In this study, middle-class children whose families had experienced economic deprivation during the depression were more achievement oriented. They were more likely to go on to higher education and were also more successful in their careers than noneconomically deprived children.

Thus, coping as a developmental process deserves systematic investigation. In a certain sense, this is an extension of the process approach to stress and coping taken by Lazarus and Folkman (1984). In

---

[2]Hobfoll (1989) has recently presented a cognitive theory of stress and coping in which coping is considered as consisting of conscious decisions concerning the expenditure of resources in stressful situations. Although resources may well be expended in coping with stress, they may also be acquired.

a process study, one examines the unfolding of a stressful episode and the attendant coping efforts over a short span of time. A life-span developmental approach tracks the effects of multiple stressful episodes in terms of relative losses and gains in coping resources during a long span of time.[3]

Aldwin and Stokols (1988) specified three developmental trajectories that could theoretically occur as a result of coping with stress based on Maruyama's (1963) modified version of systems theory. In Maruyama's model, two types of feedback mechanisms are possible, deviation countering and deviation amplification. Aldwin and Stokols hypothesized that both types of feedback may be in effect in examining the long-term effects of coping. With deviation countering, the adaptational processes return to baseline. With deviation amplification, initially small changes, whether positive or negative, can be amplified, however, and increases or decreases in adaptational resources can be seen.

Figure 4.1 demonstrates this model. First, individuals could develop increasing vulnerabilities over the life-span (the descending line). That is, through adverse experiences with stress, people may become more emotionally frail, develop negative expectancies for control, and perhaps develop serious mental health problems. Second, there could be a form of homeostasis (the middle line in Figure 4.1). Individuals may return to their initial level of functioning after stressful episodes, and exhibit little change in their adaptive capacities, either positive or negative. Finally, individuals may develop increasing resources during the life-span that more than offset any stress-related losses (the top line in Figure 4.1).

Note the assumption that there is a kind of continuity across coping episodes. Individuals may change their coping strategies across situations, but there is nonetheless an accumulation of vulnerabilities and resources, which may generalize across situations. Baltes (1987) referred to a very similar phenomenon when he depicted development in adulthood as a trade-off of losses and gains.

The construct of increases in vulnerability parallels Seligman's (1975) construct of learned helplessness, whereas homeostasis is the outcome most commonly proposed by stress researchers such as Selye (1956). The construct of increases in resources is similar to Epstein's (1983) construct of stress inoculation, although it has

[3]I am indebted to my colleague, Dr. Avron Spiro III, for this observation.

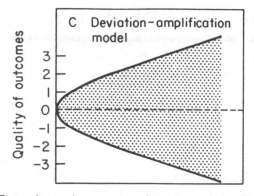

Time following onset of initial negative event

FIGURE 4.1 Temporal model of the long-term effects of stress and coping on adaptation across the lifespan. (From "The Effects of Environmental Change on Individuals and Groups: Some Neglected Issues in Stress Research" by C. Aldwin and D. Stokols, 1988, *Journal of Environmental Psychology*, 8, p. 66. Copyright 1988 by Academic Press. Reprinted by permission.

broader ramifications. Stress inoculation assumes that, through experience, individuals will no longer perceive a once stressful stimulus as threatening. An increase in resources, however, assumes that the individual has gained something that may generalize across situations.

Obviously, these are idealized trajectories, and the course of developmental change in adaptation over the life-span is undoubtedly much rougher, with plateaus, temporary setbacks, peaks, and nadirs. Nonetheless, it is interesting that these three trajectories emerged in a longitudinal study of psychological symptoms. Aldwin, Spiro, Levenson, & Bossé (1989) tracked individual change in symptoms during a 20-year period in more than 2,000 men by generating regression lines, or slopes, for each respondent. More than a third of the sample had slope coefficients of 0—that is, they demonstrated no change in psychological symptoms over time, corresponding to the middle line in Figure 4.1. More than half the sample showed only modest increases or decreases. Less than 10% of the sample showed definite decreases or increases in symptoms (e.g., greater than 1 SD above the mean).

Why these respondents changed, or did not change, in the number of psychological symptoms they reported over time is a matter of speculation. The instrument used, the Cornell Medical Index (Brodman, Erdmann, & Wolff, 1956) may not have been very sensitive to change. What change did occur may reflect objective changes in circumstances (e.g., health declines), or it may reflect the unfolding of personality predispositions over the life course. Whether or not symptom change and stability reflect stress and coping processes is unknown. Coping is a relatively new area of study, and comparable longitudinal data on stress and coping processes do not exist. A first step is to examine the relationship between stress, coping, and age.

STRESS AND COPING IN AGING CONTEXT

Depending on how the term *age* is defined, the effects of age on stress and coping processes can be roughly divided into three categories (Aldwin, 1991). First, if aging is understood as a biological process, then age may have an indirect effect on coping strategies, e.g., through the increase in health problems associated with aging. The types of problems the elderly face are often health-related problems, both in terms of their own health and in terms of the health of others in their network. Thus, they may be more likely than younger adults to be bereaved or suffer the loss of close friends and relatives.

Second, aging can also be understood in terms of cohort differences. There may be historical influences on the present population of older adults that affect their choice of coping strategies. For example, among the current elderly cohort there may be a greater reluctance to admit to psychological problems and instead substitute physical complaints.

Third, aging can also be understood in terms of intrinsic (e.g., psychological) developmental processes. Vaillant's (1977) hypothesized shift from immature or neurotic defensive styles in young adulthood to mature coping styles in midlife is one example of an intrinsic developmental process. Note that intrinsic processes can be regressive instead of developmental, as in Gutmann's (1974) hypothesized shift from active to passive mastery styles.

These intrinsic developmental processes may be better understood in terms of experience. As people age, they are exposed to a large variety of problems, and, it is hoped, through this process come to learn which types of coping strategies are generally ineffective and which types can achieve their goals in particular situations. They may also develop vulnerabilities or self-limiting adaptational styles (e.g.,

Lowenthal, Thurnher, & Chiriboga, 1975). In general, however, through experience people may increase their coping repertoire and become more able to cope successfully with difficulties.

Balanced against this increase in repertoire, however, is the fact that energy levels decrease with age. To borrow again from Baltes (1987), appraisal and coping in later life may be geared toward minimizing energy expenditure—using fewer but more effective strategies, for example.

EMPIRICAL STUDIES

Aldwin (1990) recently examined the relationship of age to the stress and coping process using a sample of 238 men and women aged 18 to 78 years who were contacted via a mail survey. The data set included measures of stress appraisals and coping processes, the revised Ways of Coping Scale (Aldwin & Revenson, 1987; Folkman, Lazarus, Dunkel-Schetter, DeLongis & Gruen, 1986). The study focused on two coping strategies, instrumental action, a problem-focused strategy referring to active attempts to manage the situation, and escapism, an emotion-focused strategy that uses wishful thinking, alcohol, drugs, or sleep to avoid the situation. Problems were also coded to indicate whether they related to health, because the higher frequency of coping episodes related to health problems among older adults may have affected the types of coping strategies they reported.

Five-point questions were also asked concerning attributions of responsibility for the occurrence of the problem and for its management, as suggested by Brickman et al. (1982). Also included was an efficacy appraisal—for example, how well the respondent thought he or she had handled this particular problem (Aldwin & Revenson, 1987). The outcome measure was the Center for Epidemiological Studies–Depression (CES-D) (Radloff, 1977), which assesses depressive symptoms.

First, a general model of the stress and coping process was constructed, using path analysis to estimate relations among stress appraisals, attributions of responsibility, the two coping strategies, perceived efficacy, and depression. These variables related to one another much as cognitive theorists such as Lazarus & Folkman (1984) and Brickman et al. (1982) have suggested. Namely, both appraisals of stress and attributions of control affected how individuals coped with problems. The more stressful the situation, the more respondents reported using escapism. Respondents who perceived that they were responsible for the management of the problem reported using more instrumental action, whereas those who perceived that they were less responsible reported using more escapism. The more instrumental action was used, the more people were likely to report that they handled the situation well and, consequently, the lower the rate of depressive symptoms.

We then added aging to the model and a variable indicating whether or not the coping episode was related to a health problem (see Figure 4.2). Despite the association between age and whether or not the respondents were coping with health problems, there was a negative coefficient between age and stress appraisals. Even controlling for health problems and stress level, age was negatively related to both attributions of responsibility. In other words, the older adults were disclaiming responsibility for the occurrence of their problems and, to a lesser extent, for the management of their problems. According to the model, this should affect their coping behavior and lead to poorer outcomes. Examining the effects of age on coping strategy use, there was an independent and negative effect of age on escapism

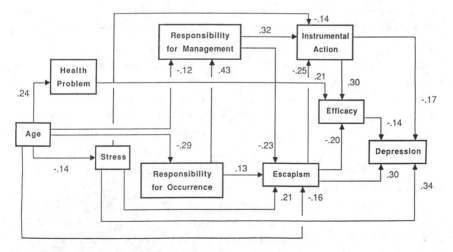

FIGURE 4.2 Model of the effects of age on the stress and coping process. From "Does Age Affect the Stress and Coping Process? Implications of Age Differences in Perceived Control" by C. Aldwin, 1991, *Journal of Gerontology*, *46*, 174–180. Reprinted by permission.

(beta $= -.16$), and no independent effects on instrumental action. In other words, although older individuals attributed less responsibility to themselves, they reported coping in ways inconsistent with their attributions. They reported less use of escapism than younger adults and reported using levels of instrumental action similar to younger adults.

Note that there was no effect of health problems on attributions of responsibility or on the use of coping strategies. Further, coping with health problems was associated with higher levels of perceived efficacy. Health problems were apparently something that these community-residing adults felt that they could handle, and handle reasonably well.

Several developmental implications can be derived from these analyses. First, age has a profound effect on the stress and coping process. It affects the types of stressful problems experienced, attributions of control, and the types of coping strategies used.

Second, age had only indirect effects on efficacy and mental health via the stress and coping process. If the elderly reported coping with health problems (which they apparently thought they could handle), and used instrumental action rather than escapism, they reported higher levels of efficacy and lower levels of depressive symptoms. This is consistent with the developmental model discussed earlier, in which the development of resources was not simply a matter of age but rather was dependent on volitional decisions made in a stress and coping context.

Third, there is an inconsistency between attributions and coping among older adults. The elderly are less likely to say that they are responsible for either the occurrence or management of their problem, yet they cope in ways that are inconsistent with these attributions. They use just as much instrumental action as younger adults, but they are less likely to use escapism. According to the model, however, denying responsibility should be associated with the use of escapist coping strategies.

This discrepancy may be explainable in terms of the energy conservation construct noted earlier. Adolescents, who have a lot of energy, often waste a lot of it in inappropriate self-blame and guilt feelings— the classic *Sturm und Drang* of adolescents. Older adults, conversely, may avoid the energy costs of such emotional upheaval by refusing to accept responsibility, thereby avoiding self-blame and guilt, but nonetheless going ahead and doing what is necessary to manage a problem.

Thus, Baltes's (1987) construct of energy conservation and the dynamic balance between losses and gains may also be a useful developmental construct for understanding change in coping strategies and stress appraisals during the life-span. We need to document the long-term effects of stress in terms of gains and losses, operationalized as changes in resources and vulnerabilities.

In collaboration with Margie Lachman and Jackie James, we conducted interviews with 160 community residents, ranging in age from young to late adulthood. Part of the interview asked the respondents to identify "low points" in their lives, and how they coped with these problems. We asked what the long-term effects of these problems were, if there were any positive aspects or if they had learned anything, and if they could draw on resources and capabilities developed in coping with earlier problems.

Preliminary readings of the interviews to date suggest that people can identify positive aspects of recent stressful experiences. Most individuals were able to describe knowledge they had gained from coping with the most recent "low point." Often these were stated in terms of interpersonal closeness—for example, "I learned that I really needed my husband, and he needed me"; or "I discovered that I could rely on my daughter in a crisis." Sometimes the learning consisted of altering appraisal processes—for example, "I learned not to sweat the little things."

There also appeared to be continuities between coping episodes, in that individuals drew on the knowledge gained from earlier stressful episodes in their current coping efforts. For example, one woman who was assisting her adult son in recovering from a major cerebrovascular accident was able to help him in part by drawing on her knowledge of hospital procedures derived from an earlier, extremely painful time in which her alcoholic husband was dying from a brain tumor. Interestingly, some individuals acknowledged that insufficient stress earlier in life made it more difficult to cope with present problems. One high school coach whose most recent low point was his team's losing season admitted that he did not know how to handle it, in part because he himself had always been on winning teams as a student athlete. He felt at a loss because he did not have past failures on which to draw.

It appeared that our respondents took developmental implications of stress and coping episodes for granted. Few said that they had not learned anything from their recent stressful experiences, and most were able to draw on past experiences as a current coping resource. We hope from this work to develop a way to categorize the long-term effects of coping and test this categorization scheme in future research.

CONCLUSION

First, the stress and coping framework may be very helpful in exploring aspects of the process of development in adulthood. Stress is universal, and may provide a context for the development of adaptive resources and vulnerabilities through the process of coping with stressful experiences. This process is largely volitional and thus does not follow a universal path across cultures. Nonetheless, coping with stress may provide a means of developing both practical knowledge, wisdom, and the "virtues" of positive characteristics that a culture may value.

Second, one potential resource appears to be a manipulation of the appraisal process. By denying responsibility, the older adults may both distance themselves from problems and avoid guilt, self-blame, and the energy expenditures associated with emotional upheavals. By managing the problem as best they can, however, they avoid the negative consequences of denying and avoiding problems.

Third, respondents acknowledge the developmental aspects of coping with stress. They can identify knowledge gained from the process and draw on earlier experiences. Preliminary research findings suggest a continuity of coping episodes during the life-span, an accumulation of resources and vulnerabilities.

Thus, by acknowledging the developmental aspects of stress, we also recognize its potentially positive aspects. We need further research that integrates stress and coping constructs with an awareness of developmental processes to understand both the long-term effects of stress and how development occurs in adulthood.

ACKNOWLEDGMENTS

Preparation of this chapter was supported by a FIRST Award from the National Institute on Aging (AG07465) and the Veterans Administration Medical Research Services. I would like to thank Professors Michael R. Levenson and Avron Spiro III for their helpful comments on earlier drafts of this chapter.

REFERENCES

Aldwin, C. (1986, May). *Cultural influences on the stress process*. Paper presented at the international symposium on "Manejo del stress: Implicaciones biologicas, psicolsocialies & clinicals." Mexico: Ensenada.

Aldwin, C. (1990). The Elders Life Stress Inventory: Egocentric and nonegocentric stress. In M. A. P. Stephens, S. E. Hobfall, J. H. Crowther, & D. L. Tennenbaum (Eds.), *Stress and coping in later-life families* (pp. 49–69). New York: Hemisphere.

Aldwin, C. (1991). Does age affect the stress and coping process? Implications of age differences in perceived control. *Journal of Gerontology: Psychological Sciences, 46,* 174–180.

Aldwin, C., & Revenson, T. (1985). Cohort differences in stress, coping and appraisal. *The Gerontologist, 25,* 66.

Aldwin, C., & Revenson, T. A. (1987). Does coping help? A re-examination of the relationship between coping and mental health. *Journal of Personality and Social Psychology, 53,* 337–348.

Aldwin, C., Spiro, III, A., Levenson, M. R., & Bossé, R. (1989). Longitudinal findings from the Normative Aging Study: I. Does mental health change with age? *Psychology and Aging, 4,* 295–306.

Aldwin, C., & Stokols, D. (1988). The effects of environmental change on individuals and groups: Some neglected issues in stress research. *Journal of Environmental Psychology, 8,* 57–75.

Baltes, P. (1987). Theoretical propositions of life-span developmental psychology: On the dynamics between growth and decline. *Developmental Psychology, 23,* 611–626.

Blanchard-Fields, F., & Robinson, S. L. (1987). Age differences in the relation between controllability and coping. *Journal of Gerontology, 42,* 497–501.

Brandtstädter, J., Krampen, G., & Heil, F. (1986). Personal control and emotional evaluation of development in partnership relations during adulthood. In M. Baltes & P. Baltes (Eds.), *The psychology of control and aging* (pp. 265–296). Hillsdale, NJ: Erlbaum.

Brickman, P., Rabinowitz, V. C., Karuza, Jr., J., Coates, D., Cohn, E., & Kidder, L. (1982). Models of helping and coping. *American Psychologist, 37,* 368–384.

Brodman, K., Erdmann, A. J., & Wolff, H. G. (1956). *Cornell Medical Index-Health Questionnaire*. New York: Cornell-University Medical College.

Dienstbier, R. A. (1989). Arousal and physiological toughness: Implications for mental and physical health. *Psychological Review, 96,* 84–100.

Elder, Jr., G. (1974). *Children of the Great Depression: Social change in life experience*. Chicago: University of Chicago Press.

Epstein, S. (1983). Natural healing processes of the mind: Graded stress inoculation as an inherent coping mechanism. In D. Meichenbaum & M. E. Jaremko (Eds.), *Stress reduction and prevention* (pp. 39–66). New York: Plenum.

Erikson, E. H. (1950). *Childhood and society*. New York: Norton.

Erikson, E. H. (Ed.). (1978). *Adulthood: Essays*. New York: Norton.

Erikson, E. H., Erikson, J. M., & Kivnick, H. Q. (1986). *Vital involvement in old age*. New York: Norton.

Featherman, D. L., & Lerner, R. M. (1985). Ontogenesis and sociogenesis: Problematics for theory and research about development and socialization across the lifespan. *American Sociological Review, 50,* 659–676.

Felton, B., & Revenson, T. (1987). Age differences in coping with chronic illness. *Psychology and Aging, 2,* 164–170.

Folkman, S., Aldwin, C., & Lazarus, R. (1981). *Locus of control, cognitive appraisal, and coping*. Paper presented at the annual meeting of the American Psychological Association, Los Angeles.

Folkman, S., Lazarus, R. S., Dunkel-Schetter, C., DeLongis, A., & Gruen, R. (1986). The dynamics of a stressful encounter: Cognitive appraisal, coping, and encounter outcomes. *Journal of Personality and Social Psychology, 50,* 992–1003.

Folkman, S., Lazarus, R. S., Pimley, S., & Novacek, J. (1987). Age differences in stress and coping process. *Psychology and Aging, 2,* 171–184.

Gatz, M., Siegler, I., George, L., & Tyler, F. (1986). Attributional components of locus of control: Longitudinal, retrospective, and contemporaneous analyses. In M. Baltes & P. Baltes (Eds.), *The psychology of control and aging* (pp. 237–263). Hillsdale, NJ: Erlbaum.

Gutmann, D. L. (1974). Alternatives to disengagement: The old men of the Highland Druze. In R. A. LeVine (ed.), *Culture and personality: Contemporary readings* (pp. 232–245). Chicago: Aldine.

Haan, N. (1978). *Coping and defending: Processes of self-environment organization*. New York: Academic Press.

Henry, W. E., & Neugarten, B. (1955, April). *Affective complexity and role perspection: Some suggestions for the study of adult personality*. Paper presented at the Conference on Research on Psychological Aspects of Aging. National Institute of Mental Health, Bethesda, MD.

Hobfoll, S. (1989). Conservation of resources: A new attempt at conceptualizing stress. *American Psychologist, 44,* 513–524.

Inkeles, A., & Smith, D. H. (1974). *Becoming modern: Individual change in six developing countries*. Cambridge: Harvard University Press.

Irion, J. C., & Blanchard-Fields, F. (1987). A cross-sectional comparison of adaptive coping in adulthood. *Journal of Gerontology, 42,* 502–504.

Lachman, M. E. (1986). Locus of control in aging research: A case for multidimensional and domain-specific assessment. *Psychology and Aging, 1,* 34–40.

Lazarus, R. S., & Folkman, S. (1984). *Stress, appraisal, and coping.* New York: Springer.

Loevinger, J. (1977). *Ego development: Conceptions and theories.* San Francisco: Jossey-Bass.

Lowenthal, M. F., Thurnher, M., & Chiriboga, D. (1975). *Four stages of life: A comparative study of women and men facing transitions.* San Francisco: Jossey-Bass.

Maruyama, M. (1963). The second cybernetics: Deviation-amplifying mutual causal processes. *American Scientist, 51,* 164–179.

McCrae, R. R. (1982). Age differences in the use of coping mechanisms. *Journal of Gerontology, 37,* 454–460.

Moos, R. H., & Schaefer, J. A. (1986). Life transitions and crises: A conceptual overview. In R. H. Moos (Ed.), *Coping with life crises: An integrated approach* (pp. 28–33). New York: Plenum.

Muhlenkamp, A., Gress, L., & Flood, M. (1975). Perception of life change events by the elderly. *Nursing Research, 24,* 727–731.

Paykel, E. S. (1983). Methodological aspects of life event research. *Journal of Psychosomatic Research, 27,* 341–352.

Pearlin, L., & Schooler, C. (1978). The structure of coping. *Journal of Health and Social Behavior, 19,* 2–21.

Radloff, L. (1977). The CES-D Scale: A self-report depression scale for research in the general population. *Applied Psychological Measurement, 1,* 384–401.

Reynolds, D. (1976). *Morita psychotherapy.* Berkeley: University of California Press.

Rodin, J. (1986). Health, control, and aging. In M. Baltes & P. Baltes (Eds.), *The psychology of control and aging* (pp. 139–165). Hillsdale, NJ: Erlbaum.

Sands, J. D., & Parker, J. (1980). A cross-sectional study of the perceived stressfulness of several life events. *International Journal of Aging and Human Development, 10,* 235–241.

Seligman, M. (1975). *Helplessness: On depression, development, and death.* San Francisco: Freeman.

Selye, H. (1956). *The stress of life.* New York: McGraw-Hill.

Silverman, M., Eichler, A., & Williams, G. (1987). Self-reported stress: Findings from the 1985 National Health Interview Survey. *Public Health Reports, 102,* 47–53.

Vaillant, G. (1977). *Adaptation to life.* Boston: Little, Brown.

Wallace, A. F. C. (1970). *Culture and personality* (2nd ed.). New York: Random House.

White, R. W. (1974). Strategies of adaptation: An attempt at systematic description. In G. Coelho, D. Hamburg, & J. Adams (Eds.), *Coping and adaptation* (pp. 47–68). New York: Basic Books.

PART II
Diversity and Adaptation to Stress

There has been a plethora of literature regarding the effects of stress and its impact on health and disease processes without any special consideration given as to how these factors operate among elderly persons. Moreover little is known as to how elderly persons respond and adapt to the strains that come from everyday living encounters. This section of the book discusses the diversity and adaptation of aged persons to stress and the aging person's response to a variety of stresses. Stressors such as unexpected loss, extreme trauma, and ethnic and racial parameters all may interact to either reduce the older adult's experience or perception of stress or add to it. The authors all seem to agree that there is considerable diversity in the stress adaptation processes that occur in old age.

Pearlin and Mullan address loss as one of the major life circumstances that produces stress, because losses inevitably increase as one ages. The loss of health, vigor, and the ability to perform activities of daily living perpetuate the daily stress and strains encountered by older adults. Pearlin and Mullan analyze conditions of loss, compensability and reversibility of loss, and the risks associated with advanced age and loss. Their chapter begins with an overview of the approaches used to study age and stress. They make an appeal to consider methodological issues, and caution against positing spurious, erroneous, and exaggerated conclusions about the relationship between age and stress that has emerged from previous research.

In the following chapter Lieberman describes limitations of a psychological stress model used in the study of widowhood. Many elderly women lose their spouses and consequently are faced with stress brought about by the loss. Lieberman discusses the concept of coping and how social support can be used to explain variations in emotional responses to stress and how aged persons manage problems of adaptation. Lieberman presents examples from several of his research studies on loss and bereavement as illustrations. According to Lieberman stressful life events are complex, multifaceted experiences that contain multiple meanings.

The next chapter focuses on the impact of extreme stress conditions on aged persons, the opposite of daily stress and strains. Boaz Kahana discusses late-life response to extreme stress experiences of prisoners of war, and victims of the Holocaust and natural disaster, classifies types of extreme stress relevant to aging, and examines late-life adaptation and its relationship to the aged person's response to earlier problems. He reports on two research studies examining the effects and response of older adults to extreme stress conditions, making comparisons between those who have adapted well and those who have made poor adjustments.

In the last chapter, Hubbard concentrates on racial, ethnic, and health status issues that may affect adaptation to stress in the aged. He discusses some critical issues regarding clinical and research perspectives on the relationship between stress and health in minority aged adults. Hubbard challenges the accuracy of stress instrumentation used with minority elderly persons and contends that the instruments as designed do not fully assess the problem of psychological stress experienced by the aged minority. He calls for studies that will help us understand what stress means to different cohorts of aged persons as well as the consideration of different racial and ethnic factors.

5

Loss and Stress in Aging

Leonard I. Pearlin and Joseph T. Mullan

Historically it has been assumed that there is a rough linear relationship between age and stress: As people get older, they increasingly encounter stressful life conditions. Although this assumption is less widely held now than in the past, several common observations of the aging process seem to support it. First, bodies change with age: They do less than they once did and with greater effort; viewed against the cultural ideals of the society, beauty—if it was ever possessed—slips from our countenances. On top of this, displacement from roles and statuses accelerates with age, presumably leaving gaping holes in the lives of people who come to feel alienated and unanchored. In short, aging brings loss with it, and loss can be a bitter and stressful pill. The problem with these assumptions and observations is that they are not fully substantiated by research findings. Although the loss of roles and statuses certainly accelerates with age, age and stress do not occur in lockstep.

One major body of evidence for this contention can be drawn from our own large-scale study of stress in a community population of adults up to the age of 65 years. When this population is divided into young adults (up to 35 years), middle-aged (36–55 years), and older adults (55 years and older), we find that indicators of stress—such as depression and anxiety—are most prominent among the young adults and least so among the oldest segment of this sample (Pearlin & Lieberman, 1979). If the sample included older people, we suspect that stress would be seen to increase among the oldest old as their functional capacities and health decline. In adulthood, then, there is probably a U-shaped curve reflecting the relationship of age and stress, with the youngest and the very oldest exhibiting most stress. In any event, we can assert that there is no straight ascending line of stress, going from the youngest adult to the oldest.

How, then, did we come to believe that aging is inherently stressful? There are two major reasons, we believe. One concerns the ways we have studied age and stress, and the other how we think about loss, what creates it, and what its effects are. We shall discuss each of these in turn.

APPROACHES TO STUDY OF AGE AND STRESS

Over the years, the study of the life-span has become highly special-ized. Scholars who study infancy or adolescence are not the same as those who study the old or the very old. Perhaps there is some good sense underlying this division of labor, but it has had some negative consequences, at least for our understanding of the relationship of age and stress across the life-span. First of all, of course, it has created a barrier to the development of a theoretical orientation that cuts across life stages or age ranks. Along with this, a sense is created that each age group is so very special that it alone experiences life circumstances that are stressful (Pearlin, 1980a).

The attention given in recent years to people at midlife (e.g., Gould, 1978; Levinson, Darrow, Klein, Levinson & McKee, 1978) illustrates the point that we wish to make. Essentially, this attention focuses solely on people in the midyears, excluding those younger or older. In their interviews with people in this age group, researchers discovered that some of the middle aged faced difficult questions, decisions, and challenges about their pasts and futures. It was an easy step to go from this information to the conclusion that midlife is a period of *Sturm und Drang*, crises, and transformations.

No one can doubt that as middle-aged people change and grow, many face critical decision points and anguish. What can be doubted is the basis for characterizing it as *the* difficult period of life, leave alone *a* period of growth, change, or crises. If the research, what there has been of it, were more comparative and less exclusively focused on a particular age group, it would have been seen that change and crises occur across the entire life span, and that they are actually more likely to be experienced by young adults than middle-aged or older people. During the 20s and 30s, there is a great deal of entry work, with people acquiring new roles and statuses. Marriage, parenthood, struggles for housing and an economic foothold are all taking place within a relatively compressed period, making midlife appear quiescent by comparison. Young adults, of course, are on the upward climb toward mature social roles; consequently, even as they endure their mounting challenges, they may enjoy the sense that they are moving toward beckoning opportunity. The possible optimism with which they may view the future notwithstanding, however, the realities of life for many young adult individuals are quite difficult.

The major point we wish to convey here is that the methods of our research in gerontology and human development and the basis on which assumptions are occasionally made can lead us to somewhat erroneous and exaggerated conclusions about the connection between age and stress. These conclusions involve implicit comparisons; that is, they necessarily assert that later ages are more stressful than earlier ones. If we are to make comparative statements involving multiple age groups, however, we cannot study but one of them. To support a comparative perspective across multiple age and life-stage groups, we must include *all* these multiple groups in the design of our research.

It is also important that we do not exaggerate the importance of age by itself. No one is *only* old or *only* middle aged. One is old and male or female, with family and friends or without, economically deprived or not, living in a safe or dangerous neighborhood, and so on. Some of the social characteristics and economic resources that people possess may suppress the relevance of age qua age. That is, a very poor young person and a very poor old person may have more in common with each other than with their age peers. There are conditions of life that constitute ambient stressors, such as poverty, and to the extent that these stressors are ubiquitous and impervious to age, they limit the association between age and stress.

The implication of this observation for our studies of age and stress is rather clear and simple: age must always be examined in conjunction with conditions that may result in stress. To the extent that these conditions are found more in one age group than another, then a connection can be claimed for an association between age and stress. It is important, however, to distinguish age-related stresses from stressful conditions that may affect people of different ages.

In sum, two methodological caveats cast a cloud over our efforts to identify the associations between age and stress. One is that past efforts have often been insufficiently comparative, leading to erroneous but popularized conclusions about the relative stressfulness of a particular age or life stage. Second, and related, it must be recognized that in and by itself, *age* is not stressful, unless, perhaps, because of its negative symbolic meaning in our society. Most typically, it is the conditions associated with age that result in stress. Age is a surrogate for many conditions and circumstances, and by itself explains little of anything. What needs to be done, consequently, is to identify the conditions associated with age that might be stressful. In doing this, however, it must be recognized that within age groups there may be considerable diversity in whether or not people are actually exposed to stressful conditions. That is, among people of the same age, there is considerable variation in many conditions associated with stress, such as poverty or ill health. Shared chronological age, therefore, is not necessarily accompanied by shared stressful conditions of life.

This is not to deny, of course, that there are stressful conditions associated with age. For example, young adults do not yet have to be concerned with such issues as the dissolution of their children's marriages or serious illness of grandchildren or the cognitive deterioration of spouses. It may also be that midlife, though not particularly stressful overall, does occasionally bring with it the need for individuals to review their accomplishments and confront the limitations of their earlier dreams. If midlife is not the time of loss, it may nevertheless be a time for contemplating the *threat* of loss. Later years, for their part, are when people may actually have to face the losses that were only feared in middle age. We have more to say about this later. The point to be underscored in these speculations, however, is that age itself is not stressful; certain conditions associated with age may be, but even those conditions do not necessarily uniformly impinge on the lives of people of the same age. Moreover, we shall see that some of the age-related conditions commonly thought to be stressful are often not.

CONDITIONS OF LOSS

As noted, the early portions of the life course are characterized by entry into new statuses and roles, and the latter parts are more marked by exits. The last of our children leave home, we are no longer engaged in a paid occupation, loved ones begin to die, and so on. Perhaps, as has been cogently argued (Rosow, 1985), the more we become separated from institutional roles and social attachments, or the more the meaningful substance of these attachments is depleted, the less the society at large values us. Anyway one looks at it, loss is not good; it can involve the pain of broken attachments to loved objects and activities; cruelly, loss as often evokes contempt as compassion for the dispossessed. To the extent that movement into old age entails mounting loss, it would seem inevitable that the aging and the aged cannot escape a fate of steadily intensifying stress. We certainly do not wish to challenge the potency of loss or its presence in the aging process. What does need to be questioned, however, is the basis for judging whether or not people experience loss.

We have indicated that loss is assumed to occur in instances of life-course transitions that entail the yielding of a role, status, activity, or relationship. It is our contention, however, that loss cannot be judged solely on the basis of whether or not such a transition has occurred. Simply put, what might appear to be a loss and, therefore, a source of stress, may not be experienced as such by the person who is in the process of exiting from the past. To gain may be better than to lose, but loss may not exist when we think we are observing it.

There are several reasons why there may be less to loss than meets the eye. First it needs to be recognized that many of the transitions that occur in the latter stages of the life course and that are assumed to entail loss are not sudden, discrete events. They typically are what we refer to as scheduled events, a term that calls attention to their links to the normative life cycle (Pearlin & Radabaugh, 1985). Because their scheduling is built into the progression of one's life cycle, however loosely, it is possible to envision or foresee these events well in advance of their occurrence. Retirement is a good example of what we are talking about in this connection. We do not usually arrive at work on a Monday only to learn that we retire on Friday. More usual, we know when we shall retire a matter of years, even decades, in advance of the actual time.

The scheduled character of these kinds of transitions means that people are able to begin preparing themselves in a way that may preclude or reduce the sense of loss that would otherwise result. This preparation represents anticipatory coping with future contingencies (Pearlin, 1980b, 1982). In the case of our retirement example, avoidance of loss by anticipatory coping might involve such diverse activities as assiduously saving money during employment, developing leisure interests and activities, expanding organizational commitments, and so on. For transitions that are sudden and eruptive, anticipatory coping is obviously less available as a cushion to loss. Such coping, however, is probably quite common in transitions that may involve very serious losses but that are previewable and open to the mental rehearsal of future conditions and personal adaptations. Examples of this preparatory coping can be seen among the close relatives of loved ones who have died after a lengthy period of being stricken with a fatal illness. In general, it seems reasonable to hypothesize that the longer individuals can foresee a future transition, the more opportunity they have to adopt behaviors to avoid or minimize loss when it does occur.

Anticipatory coping, then, is one reason why the magnitude of loss cannot be gauged solely from knowledge of a transition and of the roles, statuses, or relationships that are yielded. Another reason has to do with the quality of the role, status, or relationship that is being relinquished. We shall again take retirement as an example of this issue, because it is a transition associated with an advanced life stage. By and large, retirement has not been found to be associated with distress, probably because for each person who experiences it as a difficult transition there is another for whom it is a positive experience. What contributes to this difference, of course, is the quality of occupational life being yielded. At one extreme, it may have involved highly rewarding activities, a network of satisfying relationships, the opportunity to exercise and develop prized skills, the acquisition of status and recognition, and a sense of contributing to something worthwhile to a large collectivity. At the other extreme, work might have been routinized and deadening, it might have occurred in a harsh or indifferent authority structure that left unsatisfied one's desires for self-direction, opportunities for growth, upward mobility, and so on. For the first, retirement, especially if it is involuntary, may represent separation from a domain with which the person closely identified and to which the person's pride system was attached. For the second, retirement would mark an escape from oppression.

The point to be drawn from this example is that the transitional yielding of a role may be judged as a loss by an outside observer but not experienced as such by individuals engaged in the transition. At least for some, vacating the role will be the realization of a long-awaited dream, a chance to leave behind a difficult and onerous occupational life. The past is understandably a crucial context for shaping the meaning and impact of later experience. Role histories, as Wheaton (1990) has recently shown, need to be considered in order to make sense out of loss and stress.

Just as loss may depend on the past circumstances surrounding the vacated role, status, or relationship, it also depends on the new circumstances people face following the transition. To continue our example, the worker who looked on retirement with joy may later find that close work friends stop including him in their social plans, or people in the community do not pay him the same homage as before, or fishing every day is more boring and less fun than he had foreseen. What begins as a clear gain, therefore, may be converted by later circumstances into loss, or at least gain mixed with loss.

In the case of the death of a spouse, we see a somewhat different example of how the circumstances following a transition may influence the duration and severity of loss. There is evidence (Pearlin & Lieberman, 1979) that a chain of contingencies may be set in motion by spousal loss, the net result being an accumulation of losses. Specifically, spousal loss may lead to a loss of economic resources, status, and network. It was found that these contingent losses, which may become part of the fixed conditions of the widowed person's life, prolong and, perhaps, add to the grief and depression created by spousal loss. Unlike our hypothetical example of the retiree, therefore, in this instance future circumstances do not convert gain into loss. Instead, the initial transitional loss that accompanies spousal death is sustained and expanded by conditions created by the transition. One loss triggers other losses, and recovery from the first is impeded by the layering of other losses that continue in the form of chronic problems.

Although much more research is needed to understand better the stressful impact of transitional losses, it is evident that what makes a loss and what regulates its duration and severity is not only the fact of a transition but also the circumstances preceding and following it. This means that a transition that begins favorably may eventually turn to a loss, and one that begins as a loss may turn to a gain. Past and future circumstances also determine whether the transition will be experienced as a continuing gain or a sustained loss. What is clear is that the experience of loss cannot be judged solely on the basis of exiting from a role or relationship. When this is done, we run the inadvertent risk of either exaggerating or overlooking the losses experienced by people as they approach and enter old age. The present state of our knowledge in gerontology probably both overlooks and exaggerates loss and stress as concomitants of aging.

In attempting to trace loss from a transition, an additional complication is often encountered, one that may be referred to as indirect loss. We tend to think of transitions as the experiences of individuals, ignoring some of their important social and interactional ramifications. The consequences of a transition, however, are likely to befall not only the transiting individual but also those who are part of the individual's significant role sets. An example of what is meant here can be taken from separate interviews we conducted with a wife and her husband as part of a study of spousal support (Pearlin & McCall, 1990). The husband had retired from a middle-management position in a large corporation. He had a passion for do-it-yourself projects, and before retirement he had a list of house improvements he planned to undertake. At the time this person was interviewed, he was in the full swing of these activities and enjoying every minute of them. It was obvious that he was attacking these projects with the same zest and organizational skills that he reportedly exercised in his occupational life. His wife was a different story. During the many years of her husband's employment she understandably organized her own daytime life, one she enjoyed very much. It included lunches with friends, a regular bridge game, and a host of other discretionary activities. Her husband's retirement, his presence at home, and his expectations of her had a disruptive impact on her routines. What she previously had taken for granted she now saw slipping from her grasp. His gain from retirement, therefore, was her loss. Predictably, this created some conflict between them that was for both of them a source of distress.

This example points up that when the lives of people are closely intertwined within role sets, such as husbands and wives and parents and children, the consequences of one person's transition must necessarily affect all other parties to the role set. In this instance, one's gains were at the expense of the other's apparent loss, but this is not the only way in which gains and losses may be distributed among the members of a role set. One can imagine a situation, for example, in which the retiree experiences a loss but the spouse, happy to have the partner at home, experiences a gain. Thus, there may be many combinations, some of which can unwittingly result, as in the instance described earlier, in conflict between the members and indirectly in distress. Although the role-set reverberations of a transition are essentially unstudied, we can be certain that one person's transitional gains and losses will in one form or the other be incorporated into the experiences of all members of the role set.

In sum, loss and its stressfulness may not exist when we think it should, and it might appear when we fail to look for it. Loss depends to an appreciable extent on the meaning of the transition. Meaning, in turn, is shaped by the person's history in the role being yielded and the interpersonal relationships it entailed, and by the consequences set in motion by the transition. Some of these consequences might involve secondary losses, such as status, power, network, personal identity, or economic resources. Moreover, as we saw, stress may stem either directly from the individual's transition or indirectly from the disruptive effects of the transition on others sharing his role sets.

Putting together all of these kinds of considerations and complexities, it is understandable that the presence or absence of loss cannot be determined by assumption, no matter how reasonable the assumption appears to be. It is obvious that the issues of loss and stress in aging will be better answered by empirical information than by conjecture.

COMPENSABILITY AND REVERSIBILITY OF LOSS

We have been emphasizing that whether or not a transition is actually experienced as a loss depends on several conditions. Now we wish to suggest that when loss clearly and unambiguously does occur, the severity and duration of its impact will vary largely under the influence of two factors: its reversibility and compensability. By *reversibility* we refer to those losses that can be regained—that is, to the recapturing of relinquished roles and statuses. Not all losses are reversible, certainly; the death of a loved one with whom we enjoyed a unique relationship may defy reversal. Yet, many commonly experienced losses are amenable to reversal. Thus, the person who loses his job may succeed in finding employment at another, perhaps even better, job. The person whose spouse abandons him finds a new devoted and loving mate. The unhappy retiree reenters the labor force and reestablishes himself at his former trade. Though the pain of the initial loss may not be entirely eliminated, the ability to recapture even some of what had been lost would seem to be stress reducing.

It is interesting to speculate that the more advanced one is along the life course, the more difficult it might be to reverse previous losses. To take up our examples once again, the job loser, the divorced person, and the retiree may find it more difficult to retrieve their former statuses if they are in their 70s than in their 60s or younger. Indeed, age may be calibrated in terms of increased difficulties one encounters in attempting to reverse a loss. Thus, the reversibility of a loss depends not solely on the nature of the loss but also on the way the particular loss interacts with the age of the person who has experienced it. The impact of the same kind of loss on people of different ages, therefore, might be quite different because of the different opportunities for reversal.

Compensability is the second factor that regulates the severity and duration of loss. As we noted, some losses are difficult or impossible to reverse. Nevertheless, those that are irreversible may be compensable. That is, new or altered roles, social relationships, or activities might develop that help to compensate for those that have been lost. The newly acquired roles may not be equivalent to or strictly substitutable, but they can help to create a sense of gain that perhaps blunts loss. In the absence of research into compensable loss, we can only make assumptions about its functioning. There are many examples suggesting that compensating gains can cushion the stressful effects of losses, however. The person whose spouse dies from a fatal disease, to illustrate, may throw himself or herself into the work of organizations concerned with the disease and its victims. Personal tragedy can thus be the basis for a newfound social mission, new friends, and a boost to self-esteem. These are the kinds of compensatory gains that possibly alleviate the loss. Indeed, in some situations coping may in part be seen as a search for compensation from loss.

Obviously, much remains to be learned not only of what loss is and the conditions under which it is experienced as such, but also the conditions and qualities of loss that might help to regulate its impact. In this regard, we believe that the value placed on the lost activity or object influences the stressful effects of the loss. The more the loss is symbolically central to the self, the more severe will be its effects. We also suggest the reversibility and compensability of the loss may be influenced by its centrality. That is, the more vitally central the loss is to our priorities and values, the more difficult it may be to reverse or compensate for the loss, thus exacerbating its stressfulness.

ADVANCED AGE AND
THE HIGH RISKS OF LOSS

As we stated earlier, stress in relation to age in adulthood forms a U-shaped curve—the level of stress tends to be high among young adults and, after a decrease among the middle aged and the young-old, increases again among the old-old. There are probably many reasons for this late-life upswing, not the least of which is the increasingly looming prospect of the end of one's life. We would like to focus our attention on two general types of exigencies, both of which tend to pile up in late life and both of which are known to provoke stress in people. One of these concerns network events—that is, misfortunes that befall the people we love and whose welfare is important to us; the other concerns the misfortunes that directly befall ourselves. Although there is considerable variation among old people in their exposure to either of these circumstances, the probability of each occurring increases sharply as people advance through the ranks of the old.

Let us consider first the losses and stresses people face as a consequence of adverse network events, threats to the well-being of those who matter to us. It should be noted that these losses do not necessarily involve the kinds of transitions that we have been discussing. More often, they involve the radical transformation of roles and statuses of which people remain incumbents. Our observations about losses that stem from this source are largely drawn from our research into close relatives, primarily spouses, who are willingly but involuntarily thrust into a caregiver role as a result of their loved one being incapacitated by Alzheimer's disease. Because of increased longevity and the technological means to prolong the lives of the ill, caregiving in late life is on its way to becoming a statistically normative experience. As we shall describe, it is an experience that can leave considerable distress in its wake, especially when the incapacity involves a progressive deterioration of cognitive faculties.

Among the painful losses experienced by caregivers to husbands and wives with Alzheimer's disease are those involving cherished elements of the marital relationship. As the persona of the incapacitated individual disintegrates, so, too, do many of the central expectations and exchanges that were previously woven into the relationship. The parties to the relationship are the same, but the relationship is transformed. The fact that prized elements of the relationship disappear while one's spouse lives on may make the sense of loss all the more poignant.

The losses to which caregivers appear to be particularly sensitive include, first of all, the exchange of affection. Where caring and gestures conveying intimacy were once part of the reciprocal give and take of the relationship, they largely come to be unidirectional. The caregiver's actions toward the impaired spouse may continue to be driven by established emotional imperatives, but the caregiver is no longer the object of affection and caring as he or she probably was. The sheer reciprocity may be missed, but simply having the signs from a person who matters to you that you also matter to him or her is missed too. As could be expected, these elements of loss are related to indicators of distress, such as depressive symptomatology.

There are other losses experienced by spousal caregivers, among them the companionate or previously shared interests and activities. These can involve plans for the future that are precluded by present circumstances, the joint social participation in network relations, or the tasks that were once allocated by the household's division of labor but that now fall entirely on the shoulders of the caregiver. As difficult as these kinds of losses are to bear, probably the most serious type of loss is the *loss of self*. As caregiving comes to constitute the major part of one's life, crowding out other interests, activities, and relationships, the way one begins to think about one's self can undergo a change. Thus, to the extent that caregivers identify their own lives and fates with those of the impaired person, the more likely they are to feel that they have lost a sense of who they are and come, instead, to think of themselves as no longer being the person they once were. Along with a loss of personal identity, finally, many caregivers are susceptible to the diminishment of key self-concepts, such as mastery and self-esteem. Network losses involving important relationships, therefore, may in turn result in the loss of continuity of central elements of the self.

We might note also that losses are observed to occur outside the boundaries of the self and of the caregiving situation. Concretely, there may be economic and social losses associated with caregiving to an impaired spouse that, like those described earlier, are capable of exerting stressful consequences. Thus, reduced incomes and increased expenses may impose a concern in caregivers about the ability to sustain themselves economically in the future. The attenuation of social relations and leisure activities can also leave one feeling cut off and alienated from the worlds of which they were once a more active part.

It should be remembered that caregiving to a cognitively impaired spouse is but one example—albeit a dramatic one—of a "network event" that can trigger a host of losses. The issue to be underscored is that the likelihood that loved ones and those to whom we have strong attachments will fall into adverse circumstances increases with age. When misfortune and loss strike those who are important to us, we, too, experience misfortune and loss, even when we are not their caregivers. Of course, the same conditions that place the significant others of old people at risk also place the old people themselves at risk. When we are old, our friends and collateral relatives are no more likely to suffer misfortune than we are ourselves. When misfortune hits us directly, the losses it carries with it may be even severer than those involving others.

The direct threats and losses that the old-old experience, those not channeled through others' misfortunes, are likely to revolve around their diminished health, vigor, and mobility. We make this statement on the basis of a study led by Colleen Johnson of the oldest old, in which we are also engaged. The study involves 150 people 85 years and older who are independently living in the community. In addition to the losses that originate in their networks, this group reports considerable difficulty in managing the requirements and logistics of their daily lives because of problems of physical health. The Johnson study is still under way, and the findings are preliminary; however, it is evident that problems such as aching joints, painful feet, and general weakness and frailty are steady reminders of a lost past in which the body had performed mundane tasks that are now so difficult to execute.

One of the remarkable features of this select group of oldest old is their creative ability to live within the constraints of their reluctant and complaining bodies. Nevertheless, the loss of health and strength, which might have insidiously surfaced over many years, are difficult and irreversible circumstances. As difficult as they are in their own right, however, these kinds of limitations and losses come to stand for a more encompassing loss: the ability to control and master one's own life as one would like. Although we suggested earlier that scheduled life-course transitions may entail less loss than is ordinarily assumed, it would be difficult to exaggerate the loss of mastery as a powerful source of stress.

There are modes of coping with this kind of loss that can be discerned from the interviews with the oldest old. Basically, these coping efforts involve the realignment of priorities and the redefinition of aspirations such that the areas of life that are now beyond direct control are seen as less important or less central than those that can still be manipulated. These coping efforts notwithstanding, it is not possible to escape from the awareness that it is now necessary to rely on others for very quotidian needs that one could previously satisfy by one's own minimal effort. Reliance on others, we might note in passing, cannot be taken for granted by all of the oldest old. It usually depends on the possession of economic resources, and the physical proximity and willingness of family members. Moreover, family assistance must be given with sensitivity if the old person's sense of autonomy and independence is to be sustained. Without such sensitivity, any remaining vestiges of mastery and control are likely to be eliminated entirely. When this unfortunate state is reached, the ultimate loss is likely to occur: the loss of the desire to go on with life.

CONCLUSION

Perhaps the most salient point to be drawn from this chapter is that in their daily lives people are exposed to myriad stressful conditions and experiences. Most of these are not randomly distributed in the population; instead, they unequally befall people in different structural locations. Thus, some conditions are more likely to impinge on women than men, or more on the poor than on the rich, and still others more on one age group than another. Overall, however, the distribution of stressors by age is probably less marked than by other structural arrangements, such as gender and economic position. It is only when we reach the uppermost reaches of the age ranks that age, loss, and stress link arms closely.

This assessment is partially based on our judgment that some of the transitions that increase with age are less a source of stress than ordinarily thought, despite the fact that these transitions typically involve manifest loss. What is manifest loss to the observer, however, may not be experienced as loss by the aging individual. The experience of loss, first of all, depends on the nature of the role, the activities, or the relationship being left behind. We may assume that in general the more positively attached one was to them, the greater the likelihood that yielding will then be experienced as a stressful loss. What needs to be recognized, of course, is that the quality and intensity of attachments to the past vary considerably among those engaged in the transition.

Second, the experience of loss depends somewhat on the scope of the loss. For example, if one is widowed or retired, more may be lost than the loved person or the pleasures of being a husband or wife. One may also lose respect and recognition, economic resources, friends and other social ties, and—perhaps most important—a sense of their own identity. Thus, precisely what and how much the transition sweeps up in its path also influences whether or not it will be experienced as loss.

Third, and related to the preceding, transitions are best understood both as moving away from former circumstances and moving into circumstances newly created by the restructuring of one's life. Occupational retirement, for example, does not necessarily leave a void that work once occupied. For many, new activities and interests fill that life space, a process that might anticipatorily begin even in advance of the transition. Of course, if these new activities are unrewarding, then we can expect that the loss experienced from the transition will remain or grow.

Finally, not all transitions can be treated as equivalent. Thus, some experienced losses may be reversible, such as may be witnessed in the case of the unhappy retiree who reenters the labor force. By contrast, the death of a loved one is not reversible. Nonreversible losses may be compensable, however. That is, activities, relationships, or commitments may surface that act to counterbalance the distress created by the loss. As a general proposition, we suggest that losses that occur in highly valued areas of life and that are neither reversible nor compensable are the most stressful, other things being equal.

It is among the old-old that the clearest connections can be observed involving age, loss, and stress. Perhaps nothing is more stressful in the upper reaches of the age structure than the necessity to confront one's own shrinking autonomy and mastery. The inexorable loss of these cherished elements is often forced into recognition by general frailty or health problems that limit stamina and strength. The loss of personal mastery is probably all the more bitter a pill by virtue of the fact that among the old-old it is likely to be both irreversible and noncompensable.

Although we are on some fairly certain grounds with respect to our knowledge of age and stress, a note of suggestiveness and speculation can be discerned throughout this chapter. This is as it should be, for much remains to be learned, and some of what we think we know needs to be questioned. The best way to go about this learning task, we believe, is by designing research that allows comparisons across the life course, that involves people who are representative of the diverse structural segments of the society, and that employs conceptual frameworks that provide a meaningful guide to inquiry and interpretation. Until a body of research is developed that meets these criteria, we must look at aging, loss, and stress with a proper degree of tentativeness.

REFERENCES

Gould, R. L. (1978). *Transformations: Growth and change in adult life.* New York: Simon & Schuster.

Levinson, D. J., Darrow, C. N., Klein, E. B., Levinson, M., & McKee, B. (1978). *The seasons of a man's life.* New York: Knopf.

Pearlin, L. I. (1980a). Life strains and psychological distress among adults. In N. J. Smelser & E. H. Erikson (Eds.), *Themes of work and love in adulthood* (pp. 174–192). Cambridge, MA: Harvard University Press.

Pearlin, L. I. (1980b). The life cycle and life strains. In H. M. Blalock, Jr. (Ed.), *Sociological theory and research: A critical appraisal* (pp. 349–360). New York: Free Press.

Pearlin, L. I. (1982). Discontinuities in the study of aging. In T. K. Hareven & K. J. Adams (Eds.), *Aging and life course transitions: An interdisciplinary perspective* (pp. 55–74). New York: Guilford.

Pearlin, L. I., & Lieberman, M. A. (1979). Social sources of emotional distress. In R. G. Simmons (Ed.), *Research in community and mental health* (Vol. 1, pp. 217–248). Greenwich, CT: JAI Press.

Pearlin, L. I., & McCall, M. (1990). Occupational stress and marital support: A description of microprocesses. In J. Eckenrode & S. Gore (Eds.), *Stress between work and family* (pp. 39–60). New York: Plenum.

Pearlin, L. I., & Radabaugh, C. (1985). Age and stress: Processes and problems. In B. B. Hess & E. W. Markson (Eds.), *Growing old in America: New perspectives on old age* (pp. 293–308). New Brunswick, NJ: Transaction Books.

Rosow, I. (1985). Status and role change through the life cycle. In R. H. Binstock & E. Shanas (Eds.), *Handbook of aging and the social sciences* (2nd ed., pp. 62–93). New York: Van Nostrand Reinhold.

Wheaton, B. (1990). Life transitions, role histories, and mental health. *American Sociological Review, 55,* 209–223.

6

Limitations of Psychological Stress Model: Studies of Widowhood

Morton A. Lieberman

The social and behavioral sciences have, in the past several decades created a new growth industry, stress studies. Despite important conceptual variations and their associated controversies, a general stress model remains solidly entrenched. This model posits that life conditions or life events unleash a complex process in people, who respond as if they needed to maintain or reestablish homeostasis. Central are cognitive processes (Lazarus & Folkman, 1984) that are key to the type and intensity of subsequent response. Attention in the "general" framework is usually focused on a variety of strategies for containing the "stressor." Coping strategies and social supports are two important constructs used to explain variations in how people address the problems engendered by the stress as well as the emotional reactions elicited. The adequacy of the cognitive and behavioral sequences set in motion by the stress event or condition is evaluated by indexes measuring adaptation—mental or physical health, well-being, and role performance. Departures on these indexes in a negative direction connote failure, the absence of such departures represent successful adaptation.

My past work on the adult life cycle was structured by such a framework. In the 1960s and 1970s, Dr. Sheldon Tobin and I studied the elderly's movement from one residential setting to another. We examined two stressor models: environmental discrepancy and loss. The former provided a more parsimonious and robust explanation than did a loss-intensity framework (Lieberman & Tobin, 1983). In the 1970s and early 1980s, Dr. Leonard Pearlin and I applied a stress model to a large longitudinal random sample of adults. Stress was viewed as originating from the occurrence of life events, as well as the conditions of day-to-day life. We found that the simple equation of life transitions and subsequent adaptation is not a powerful model for examining the adult life cycle (Pearlin & Lieberman, 1978). A subsequent study (Cohler & Lieberman, 1978; 1980) of midlife and elderly ethnic elders examined the effects of "culture" on patterns of adaptation in response to stressful life circumstances. We found major cultural differences. Cultural affiliation affected successful responses to stress and the meaning of life events. (Similar events did not have the same stress affects measured by subsequent outcomes.)

These studies on environmental change and adult transitions emphasized a loss model. In all the expected linkage, albeit a relatively weak one, between loss and failures in adaptation was observed. The absence of robust associations between events and consequences was addressed by examining intervening constructs—coping strategies and available psychological resources. Similar to many preceding and subsequent research reports, this model bore fruit and served as a framework for understanding the complex linkage between stressful circumstances and adaptational success or failure. Despite such success, the frequency that some of the same studies' findings failed to fit the model raised my level of discomfort with a general stress paradigm. Several new studies, to be discussed, clearly demonstrate this concern. They also underscore how such reliance on general stress paradigm can lead to misguided attempts to be helpful to those undergoing stress.

This chapter reviews findings from several of my recent loss studies. The results call into question two commonly made assumptions. On the input side of the stress equation (the stressor) the findings suggest that the ordering of life events on a single dimension, such as the amount or intensity of loss, or the amount of change, ignore salient and impactful characteristics of life events. On the output side, data will be presented suggesting that a stress model's emphasis on adaptation based on homeostasis ignores important reactions to life events.

STUDIES OF SPOUSAL BEREAVEMENT

Consequences of Widowhood: Unanticipated Findings

Recent widows and widowers (average age, 57 years) were recruited for a controlled clinical trial to determine the efficacy of brief group psychotherapy (Lieberman & Yalom, in press). The sample, ($N = 60$) included 80% of the widows and widowers whose spouse had died in cancer wards of Stanford University Hospital. Thirty-six were randomly selected for intervention. All were interviewed at length (2–6 hours), and assessed on measure of grief, mental health, social functioning, self-image, and attitudes. We repeated these measures and interviews 1 year later.

As our research team (Drs. Yalom, Guttman, Lomeranz, and Lieberman) listened to the taped interviews, they slowly became aware (and, I would add, much too slowly for such a group of experienced clinicians) that many of the widows exhibited behaviors that demonstrated reintegration and current functioning that appeared higher than their prewidowhood levels. Expectations based on the psychology of loss would not "predict" that a substantial minority would show higher levels of both internal and external behavior patterns— "growth" within the first year of widowhood.

We initiated a formal study, using two independent raters to assess "growth" and person-situation characteristics hypothesized as linked to growth (Yalom & Lieberman, in press). We found that "growth" was orthogonal to other adaptation measures common in bereavement studies; intensity of grief, intrusive thoughts about the dead spouse, mental health, mental distress, and role functions. Some respondents rated as "high growth" at both time 1 (T1; initial interview) and at time 2 (T2; 1 year later) showed, for example, elevated depression scores. Growth describes a different way of looking at adaptation.

"Growth" is not a random event; it is linked to theoretically relevant processes. We examined the effects of spousal loss on thoughts about personal death, reexaminations of purpose in life, past regrets, and aloneness. We saw the loss of the spouse in long-term marriages as stimulating existential concerns. Widows who engaged in these explorations were more likely to show patterns of "growth" than those who did not.

These findings of a reaction pattern to loss not encompassed by a homeostatic model suggests opening up our definition about spousal loss. We need to look at widowhood not simply as loss but as a multifaceted challenge. Constructs are required that encompass the emergence of various challenges during the course of the first few years of widowhood. The tasks associated with widowhood include dealing with grief and loss, managing the role transitions from married to single status, changes in self-identity, managing social network, and, as indicated, existential dilemmas.

This view of spousal bereavement requires an examination of specific challenges and their possible orderly progression over time. It raises questions about an all-encompassing single episode.

Loss Theory and Reactions to Spousal Bereavement

It is commonly assumed that the absence of grief following bereavement represents some form of pathology (Lindemann, 1944), and that the failure to experience distress and "work through this distress" portends future difficulties. A time line describes the progression of grief, with the suggestion by some that there are formal stages through which the prototypical bereaved person must pass. This time line is frequently used to provide a guideline to the bereaved person's successful adaptation. Protracted grief is seen as a sign of pathology similar to the absence of grief. A recent review by Wortman and Silver (1987) provides some evidence to challenge these views of spousal bereavement.

I followed a sample of 239 widows (average age at the time of widowhood was 56.3 years) during 7 years. The first point of measurement was within the first 24 months of widowhood, the second a year later, and the last was 6.5 years after the initial assessment (Lieberman & Videka-Sherman, 1986).

Most bereavement studies rely on measures of the consequences of grieving for evidence of grief. I used a different approach to indexing levels and intensity of grieving by relying on phenomenological measures. Each respondent was asked to indicate how much grief they were experiencing and the frequency of intrusive thoughts about the lost spouse. Respondents who reported that they experienced no grief and did not think about their dead spouse were classified as a "no-grief" group; those reporting they experienced some grief but rarely, if ever, thought about their lost husband were classified as showing mild grief; those who indicated they experienced some grief and frequently thought about their dead husband were classified as a moderate grief group; and those who indicated a great deal of grief and were frequently preoccupied with the dead spouse were classified as showing intense grief. At T1, 12% of our sample reported no grief, 30% reported mild grief, 43% moderate grief, and 15% intense grief.

How well did this measure work? A significant linear relationship was found between the level of grief and a variety of mental health and psychological stress measures. No-grief widows at T1 were found to have the highest scores on measures of coping, mastery, self-esteem, and well-being, and the lowest scores on depression, anxiety, perceived poor health, and distress experienced with problems of widowhood. Those at high levels of grief showed a reverse pattern: low scores on coping, mastery, self-esteem, and well-being; high scores on symptoms, ill health, and distress.

We were also interested in patterns of grief over time and used this grief classification system for assessing the respondent 1 year later, T2. Four grief types were developed: (a) "no-grief" widows who showed no grief both at T1 and T2, (b) "delayed-grief" widows who at T1 showed little grief but at T2 showed moderate to intense grief, (c) "recovered-grief" widows who at T1 showed moderate to intense grief and at T2 showed no or very mild grief; and (d) "chronic-griever" widows who showed moderate to intense grief at both T1 and T2. For this last group a time dimension was added. To be classified as a chronic griever, intense level of grief had to be present for at least 2 years beyond their husband's death.

What are the consequences of these grief patterns? T2 adaptation scores (measures of mental health, positive psychological states, and roles) were adjusted for T1 using a multivariate analysis of covariance model. The best adapted were the nongrievers, widows who showed a pattern of recovery based on our grief measures showed significant improvement by T2. The delayed-grief group showed some decrements, whereas the chronic-grief group remained substantially lower on all the measures compared with all the other grief patterns. The influences of grief patterns were, however, not apparent on measures of long-term (7 years) adaptation. Our assessment of mental health, positive psychological states, measures of role, and a measure of growth adjusted either for T1 or T2 revealed no significant differences among the grief groups after 7 years.

What do our findings tell us about stress? Responses to the loss as indexed by patterns of grieving has significant consequences for adequacy of adaptation assessed within the first several years of bereavement. Expectations based on clinical studies about chronic grieving are fulfilled. The suggestions about the resolution of grief as well as the bereaved who initially avoid or deny grief (the delayed group) match our findings. The findings that the best adapted are widows who appear not to grieve does not support a loss model, however. Were the nongrievers unusual or in some way limited? We tested a hypothesis of emotional constriction by examining their level of growth. They were just as likely to show a pattern of growth as were any of the other groups of widows classified on the basis of their grief patterns. Growth was found, in a previous study (Yalom & Lieberman, 1991), to be linked to engagement in existential issues, a process that requires an introspective stance. How useful, then, is it to see widowhood simply as a loss? The findings do not support the view that the experience of loss affects all, and individual differences in reactions are explained by a complex set of "down-line" processes (e.g., coping).

Who are these women who did not experience grief? We examined a series of hypotheses based on differences in their relationship before the lost spouse, their social context, and their embeddedness in a social network providing resources. The only significant difference between these women and those who reported grief was their relationship to the dead husband. Widows who did not grieve were, before the death of the husband, less dependent on their spouse, and they showed less ambivalence as measured by current guilt and anger. In sharp contrast were the chronic grievers who showed high dependence and high ambivalence as indexed by guilt and anger. These findings may be interpreted by some as an elaborate argument suggesting that the meaning of the event was different for these two groups of widows. No evidence appeared in the study that the appraisal of the event itself, the loss, differed systematically among the grief groups. All saw it as a profound loss. What differed were their reactions. These findings about grief patterns combined with the observations on positive conse-quences of widowhood suggest that we need to carefully reexamine the framework for studying the commonest form of stress, losses.

STUDIES OF SELF-CONCEPT STABILITY AND CHANGE

The last area of empirical exploration to be reported looks at the linkages between life stress and stability of the self-image. Two studies will be reviewed: one examines a variety of life events involving loss;

the other is a study of one type of loss—spousal bereavement. The findings question the appropriateness of developing a single dimension, differing in intensity, for indexing diverse life events. I have chosen this area for investigation because of two competing views about the stability of the self-image under stress. It has been shown to be valid that, overall, there is a strong "drive" to maintain a coherent and consistent self-image despite the vagaries of external events (Rosenberg, 1979). In my work examining an elderly population under situations of high stress, observations similar to that of Rosenberg were made. Lieberman and Tobin (1983) found that the elderly, despite radical change in their environment, maintain a coherent and consistent self-image. A variety of psychological devices were used by them in maintaining their self-image despite the fact that the feedback offered by the current environment to maintain elements of the self-construct had been radically altered. We found that some elderly went to great lengths to maintain consistency—an unchanging self over time. Psychological strategies involving distortion, or denial, or the creation of mythologies were used to maintain a consistent self-image.

This apparent "drive" for self-image consistency and stability, when confronted with stress, appears to conflict with the requirements for successfully negotiating the task of widowhood. In two lives that are intertwined over the years the self-image of each of the partners takes on many of the characteristics of the other—in some sense, a "couple's" self-image. Furthermore, a major source of support for many of the self-image constructs are based on feedback from the spouse. When this feedback is suddenly removed, as it is for widows and widowers, the remaining spouse is faced with reconstructing self-image now that the person is an "I" rather than a "we," and now that many of the sources of information necessary to maintain a coherent and consistent self-image (i.e., feedback from the deceased spouse) are no longer available. On these grounds we anticipate that widows who successfully navigate the strains and challenges linked to the death of a spouse would be ones who are able to revise their self-image.

Thus, we are faced with two competing views: (a) a general stress view, supported by some empirical findings, that successful adaptation is correlated with the ability to maintain a coherent and consistent self-image despite changes in life circumstances commonly labeled stressful; and (b) our view of widowhood and its required modification of the self-image. These perspectives will be explored using empirical data from two studies: one addresses a variety of life events commonly used to index loss intensity; the other addresses self-image changes and adaptation among a group of widows. The first study represents an examination of the impact of various stressful life events on self-image change and draws on the data developed in a panel study that began with a random sample of 2,300 adults who were followed five years later. The second study examines widows in the clinical intervention trial.

Impact of Life Events and Normative Transitions on Changes in the Self

A probability sample of 2,300 adults age 18 to 65 years were studied at two points in time, separated by 4.5 years (the Chicago transition study [see Pearlin & Lieberman, 1978, for a detailed description of sampling methods]). Examined were a variety of hypotheses about the effects of stress in adult lives and the role that psychological coping strategies (Menaghan, Pearlin, Lieberman, & Mullan, 1984), as well as sources of help, both formal and informal, play in respondent's psychological and physical health (Lieberman & Glidewell, 1978). A subset of the data generated is relevant to changes in self. Respondents were asked to identify specific normative transitions and eruptive events that occurred between the T1 and T2 interviews. Included were occupational events, promotions, job changes, job losses, and exits and entries into the labor force; family events, marriage, birth of a baby, new status as a grandparent, changes in marital status, alterations in the status of the children; entrance into school, and departure from home; and family illnesses and losses through death of significant others. If any occurred between the T1 and T2 interview, respondents were asked about their level of pre-occupation or intrusiveness on their daily thoughts (frequency of thinking about the event during the past week); how much the event has changed their lives; if a positive event, the degree to which they were pleased about it; and changes in the way they feel about themselves. If the respondent indicated changes in the self, they were asked about the content of self-image changes: did they become more, less, or stay the same on eight self-image constructs: respect, distance, competency, disappointment, responsible, dependent, wise, and in control of life?

Our measure of self-concept stability and instability is different from those previously reported in the literature (Lieberman & Tobin, 1983; Mortimer, Finch, & Kumka, 1982; Rosenberg, 1979). Ordinarily stability and instability are defined using T1 and T2 correlations based on the content of the self-image. The study strategy is based on a phenomenological definition; respondents are asked whether their self-image has changed as a result of a particular event and if so to indicate the content areas of such changes.

Events differed markedly in the proportion of people who perceived changes in the self. High-perceived self-change events included divorce, 73%; job entry, 62%; job change, 44%; promotions, 41%; marriage, 39%. Low impact on the self-image events included child starting school, 15%, child leaving home, 12%; child bearing, 6%; becoming a grandparent, 12%; major decrements in health, 10%; and declines in their elderly parents, 12%.

Previously published work with the sample (Pearlin et al., 1981), found many of these events, particularly eruptive crises, had a profound but indirect effect on subsequent psychological adjustment. Perhaps more important for the present chapter was the effect of perceptual variables on subsequent outcomes. High preoccupation with a negative event led to subsequent high level of depression and frequent help seeking (Lieberman & Mullan, 1978). Perceived changes in the self and preoccupation, however, are only moderately related ($r = .27$). This suggests that these are independent appraisals by the respondent of the meaning of an event. Greater overlap was found for perceptions that events change a respondent's life and changes in the self ($r = .68$). Although moderately intercorrelated, there were important exceptions to the relationship between these perceptions. For example, changes in a person's own health between the T1 and T2 interview had a substantial impact on perceptions of life changes, but infrequently was perceived as evoking changes in self. Similarly, retirement was perceived by most as having a substantial impact on their lives but rarely led to self-changes. Some events were perceived as engendering changes in the self (such as job disruption and promotions) but not as evoking life changes.

Variations Among Participants in Perceived Self-Change

Many respondents, no matter how many or what kind of life events they experienced, did not report changes in their self-image. Most of them, however, acknowledged the impact of the event by reporting it as having changed their lives and saw the event as personally salient by stating that it was frequently on their mind even after the passage of several years. A minority of the respondents perceived the same events as having had a substantial impact on how they think about themselves. These variations in *perceived self-change* is the analytical focus.

Negative life events that involved substantial psychological losses to the respondent were selected. Included were changes to a lower standard of living, exits from the job market (demotion, firing, or layoff), changes in the status of the respondent's parents; and negative health events, hospitalizations of the respondent, their spouse, or child; and the loss, through death, of significant others. All these events have been shown, in previous research (Lieberman & Glidewell, 1978; Mullan, 1981; Pearlin & Lieberman, 1978), to have a substantial impact on subsequent mental, physical, and social functioning in T2 respondents ($N = 1106$). (See Pearlin & Lieberman [1978] for details of sample attrition of T1 and T2 respondents. Overall, the probability sample drawn at T1 was not seriously compromised.) T2 respondents were divided into those who had one or more of these loss events between T1 and T2, and those who did not; 80% had one or more loss event. There were no statistically significant differences on measures of psychological symptoms nor indexes of psychological resources (self-esteem and coping mastery) between these two groups *before* the negative event. As anticipated their psychological functioning declined (assessed at T2) subsequent to the loss event. Of those who experienced one or more loss events, 22% perceived changes in their self-image.

Subsequent analysis compared subjects who experienced similar events and reported a change of self to those who did not report changes in the self on measures of psychological function before the event (T1). Three general dimensions were examined, with T1 mental health measured by levels of anxiety and depression (Pearlin & Lieberman, 1978); self-measures, the Rosenberg Self Esteem Scale (Rosenberg, 1965) and Coping Mastery (Pearlin & Lieberman, 1978) (internal or external locus of control); and two core personality dimenisons: dominance and affiliation (Leary, 1957). The two groups (self; malleable, nonmalleable) were compared on a series of tests using their T1 scores. Respondents who perceived a change in the self were significantly more anxious before the event ($\bar{x} = 1.48$,

$\bar{x} = 1.34$); depressed ($\bar{x} = 0.51$, $\bar{x} = 0.39$); had lower self-esteem ($\bar{x} = 0.67$, $\bar{x} = 0.70$); coping mastery ($\bar{x} = 3.53$, $\bar{x} = 3.71$); and dominance ($\bar{x} = 0.07$, $\bar{x} = 0.14$) than did subjects who reported no changes in the self-image as a consequence of the event(s) (all test were $= p \leq .05$). Analyses disaggregating each specific loss event showed that the type of loss event had no effect on these reported findings; the T1 scores of those who reported self-changes after the event were less adequate when compared with subjects who experienced the same event but did not see it as changing their self-image.

Next we asked whether the total number of changes in the self-image were related to T1 scores on mental health, self-image, or personality. The previous analysis contrasted groups of people categorized by the presence or absence of self-change; here we looked at the number of self-constructs used to describe change. We tested the linear relationship, using analysis of variance, between the T1 variables and the number (from 0–7) of self-construct changes. A significant ($p \leq .001$) relationship was found between measures of mental health, self, and personality with the number of self-changes. The greater the number of constructs used to describe changes in the self, the higher T1 anxiety and depression, and the lower the mastery, self-esteem, and dominance.

Were these results affected by the directionality of self-reported change? Did people who saw life events as affecting their self-concept in a negative direction as becoming less capable, more distant, less responsible, less in control, more disappointed, less wise, more dependent, and less self-respecting systematically differ from those who reported themselves as possessing an enhanced self-image (i.e., more capable, closer, more responsible, more in control, less disappointed, wiser, and more self-respecting)? Analyses examining, separately, the number of positive and negative changes to the self were calculated. The results were similar to the previously reported findings: Respondents who reported that their self-images had changed as a result of a life event by becoming more positive still showed poorer T1 functioning on mental health, self, and dominance. As a final test of the content changes in the self-image, positive and negative ratios (number of positive versus negative constructs) were calculated for each individual. The ratio of positive to negative did not alter the previously reported results. The results are clear and unambiguous; respondents who interpret negative life events as leading to changes in their self image, no matter what the content of the self-change, showed scores reflecting poorer psychological functioning before the life event that "elicited" the self-revision compared with those who experienced the same event but saw the self as less mutable.

Study of Mid- and Late-Life Widows and Widowers

The clinical controlled trial of intervention sample previously described was used to study self-image change and stability. The self-sort questionnaire and interview was used to assess self-concept change (Lieberman & Tobin, 1983). This instrument consists of 48 interpersonal statements drawn from the Leary checklist (Leary, 1957). Respondents were asked to select items like themselves and those unlike themselves. They were then asked to indicate for those self-descriptive items currently like themselves which of the items they selected reflect new self-images within the last year (new). Similarly, they were asked to look once again at the items that were selected as not currently characteristic of themselves and to indicate which of these used to be like themselves (old). Finally, the respondent was asked to provide examples from their current life that supported their self-image. These open-ended responses were coded on a 13-point scale assessing quality of support (evidence) for self-image (Rosner, 1968). This instrument was repeated 1 year later.

The mean number of revisions of the self-image soon after widowhood (T1) was the average of 8 items (out of a theoretically possible 48 items chosen to be like the self); the average number of items chosen was slightly under 30. The mean number of self-image revisions in which the spousally bereaved saw changes in the self based on new qualities was 4.8; for characteristics that used to be like themselves but were currently unlike themselves, 3.3. Looking at the distributions, for old characteristics, 24% had none, 50% had a few (1–3) and 26% had more than 3; for new characteristics 22% had none, 26% had a few (1–3), and the remainder (52%) had more than 3. About 25% of the self-image constructs were seen as undergoing change by this group of widows and widowers.

You will recall that this group of spousally bereaved was studied at 2 points in time, T1 approximately 4 to 6 months after the death of the spouse and once again a year later. Because the widowers generally showed different response characteristics on most measures of impact and the small sample size precluded covariance procedures, they were not considered in this analysis. Twenty-two widows participated in a brief group psychotherapy intervention, the remainder ($n = 14$) were randomly selected for a nonintervention control. The small sample size makes it difficult to construct analytical statistics. Simple correlations, however, between self-change (a combined score of old plus new items) indicate directions of relationships that are quite unlike those reported in the previously described normative sample. Five dimensions were used to index reactions to spousal loss: *intensity of mourning* (self-reported level of grief, intrusive thoughts, intensity of anger, and intensity of guilt); *effectance*, the composite score of self-esteem, well-being, and coping mastery (locus of control); *symptoms of grief*, a composite measure based on depressive symptoms, anxiety symptoms, somatic symptoms, the degree to which health interferes, and the frequency of medication and alcohol abuse for mood change; a measure of *role strain* in the single role; and the *degree of stigma*.

Correlations were calculated between self-concept revisions using three scores, the number of new, old, and a total amount of self-change. These variables were correlated with the five basic outcome measures—grief, positive feelings, symptoms of grieving, role distress, and stigma. Those who had many revisions of the self-image based on both old and new had statistically significant lower grief at both T1 and T2 (average correlation $r = 0.30$). They also had lower scores on symptoms of grief, but the directions were different for those whose self-concept revisions were based on new self-constructs. These widows showed significantly lower symptoms ($r = 0.32$) compared with those who saw little change in their self-image and compared with those whose change was based on the revision of self by extruding old elements. The remainder of the outcome indicators was somewhat confusing; in contrast, our measures of effectance (coping mastery, self-esteem, and well-being), although at T1 showing a small positive relationship to self-revision, at T2, a year later, were sharply reversed ($r = 0.20$) between revisions of the self based on both new and old and positive states. In short, revisions of the self seem to lead to increased feelings of reduced self-esteem and reduced well-being. Finally, on the role measures there was a modest relationship between self-change, but again, there was a sharp difference between whether self-change was based on revisions using new elements that was unrelated to increases in role strain, whereas those widows who revise self-images by extruding previously held self-constructs showed a correlation of $r = .30$ with increased role strain.

The results are certainly only tentative and more complex than would permit a simple explanation. The finding, however, that revisions of the self-image among widows in the areas directly addressing bereavement—both the intensity of grief and the symptoms associated with grief—are more functionally and more successfully addressed by those widows who do revise the self-image. This stands in contrast to the previous findings from the normative sample in which such fluidity of self-image was associated with poor adaptation.

We do not have an adequate control group using identical measures of self-image revisions. To provide some perspective on the relationship between self-concept revisions and adaptation based on identical measures, I will briefly describe one additional study (Lieberman & Stilliger, 1990). Seventy-seven adults ranging from age 22 to 55 years (median, 33 years) were about to enter large-group awareness training, a volitional change setting in which people come because they express some dissatisfaction with their current lives and how they are living them. In such settings, the absence of changes in the self-concept might be perceived by clients as a failure. Measures of self-concept and outcome identical to those used in the widow study were used. Hierarchical regression equations revealed that both revisions of the self before the training and subsequent to the training (1 year later) were linked to decrements in both positive mental health scores and positive states. In other words, in this volitional change study where expectations would be that self-revisions were part and parcel of the expectational set for entering the change setting and would be seen as successful, those individuals who before the training or subsequent to the training did a lot of self-revision were less well adapted, a finding that parallels our observations on the normative study.

IMPLICATIONS

The analysis of reactions to spousal bereavement by two samples of women (who are not economically deprived) reveal that many widows did not follow the patterns anticipated by the application of a loss model. Unanticipated outcomes including growth in response to loss, the absence of mourning associated with excellent adaptation, and the reversal of self-concept stability when adaptation were compared with other loss life events lend support to the limitations of a loss framework.

These findings do not lead necessarily to the view that the general paradigm applied in stress studies is incorrect or even that it is not useful. Rather, they suggest that such a framework is limited. Life events, even such a powerful one as a loss of a spouse, sets off a complex chain of consequences. I have used the language of tasks or challenges to describe these consequences. Even a partial listing of these tasks served to underscore the complexity of a single event that we had labeled stressor.

The widow is faced with a major task in renegotiating her social support and social network system. The complexity of patterns in this area may perhaps best be expressed by a study addressing social supports and social networks. A recent study of social networks (Lieberman, Mullan, & Heller, 1990), using the same sample of widows cited here for the grief study, examined the social networks and sources of social support among widows. We found that those who established a mixture of new and old friends that contained other widows were much more likely to be helped, measured by adaptational success, compared with those who relied totally on their old social networks. A surprising 20% of the widows studied reconstituted a totally new social network. Judging by these findings, it seems clear that a major task facing the new widow during several years is a reconfiguration and a renegotiation of their social network.

A central issue facing the widow is moving from a self-image embedded in a long-term relationship to a self based on an "I." This is clearly a daunting task, particularly for widows from traditional marriages. This challenge can be a source of distress for many; for others, however, it appears to provide a sense of accomplishment. Such variations in response suggest that it is an aspect of spousal bereavement that needs to be studied in its own right and not subsumed under a loss rubric.

Other issues described by the label "existential" focus on the inner life of the widow, again directing our attention to examining widowhood beyond a stress paradigm. Confronting regrets not only about their marital relationship but also for undeveloped aspects of their lives, has led, for some, to growth. Dealing with a sense of aloneness provides a constant source of both distress and a potential stimulus for future progress. I am not talking here about loneliness, which represents the external social component, but the issue that seems so paramount among many of our widows in recognizing their essential aloneness despite the embeddedness in an ongoing social network made up of friends and family. In a study most recently completed, it became clear that loneliness and aloneness were quite different (as they have been conceptualized by theoreticians interested in an existential position). We found, for example, that the men we studied experienced aloneness much more intensely, or at least were less willing to tolerate the feeling generated by this state. They frequently translated this to loneliness and just as quickly appeared to find a source for assuaging the latter but not necessarily the former feeling. By the end of one year, 90% of the men we studied in the controlled clinical trial had entered into a permanent heterosexual relationship. Many of the women in that study, although dating and having accessible males, clearly were not at that point in their lives willing to again enter such a relationship. In our terms, they were more able to deal with the issue of aloneness and not convert it into feelings of loneliness that can more readily be fixed by finding a significant other.

This list of issues of tasks could be broadened, but I think my illustrations are sufficient to make a simple point: the focus on the loss, as if it were a singular event, has limited usefulness; these limits on its usefulness can perhaps be seen more clearly around spousal bereavement. It has, I think, led us to ignore the positive consequences that appear to be common for several widows. Again, the language of loss or stress does not encourage the search for the articulation of positive consequences. I think the singular event focus on spousal bereavement has also led us to overlook the fact that the emotional processes of dealing with the loss may vary greatly, and that the failure to engage in such a process is not *prima facie* evidence for pathology. Our semantics of loss have I think enabled or facilitated our ability to ignore other aspects of this complex human event. The reliance in a stress model of assessing consequences for adaptation based on a homeostatic assumption clearly limits the appropriate search for other concepts. Finally, I think a loss framework in an overinclusive construct in which we have taken as a field a series of discrete—and I believe qualitatively different—events, and connected them, enables us to draw broad pictures but ignore important differences and linkages between an event and the consequences of such events for the future viability of the people experiencing such events.

I believe that the findings reported in this chapter underscore the restrictions that the general stress theory places in understanding major life events. Such events are complex and contain multiple meanings and challenges for the person. It is not simply an issue of individual difference and reactions to a common event. Rather, the event itself is multifaceted, and differences observed in consequences or reactions to the events must be linked to aspects of the event as well as how the person interprets the events, or the types of resources and coping strategies they bring to bear on the event. We need to understand what aspects of events at what time subsequent to events are being responded to and reacted to before we can understand variations both among people and within the same person over time.

REFERENCES

Cohler, B., & Lieberman, M. A. (1978). Ethnicity and personal adaptation. *International Journal of Group Tensions, 7*(2), 20–41.

Cohler, B. J., & Lieberman, M. A. (1980). Social relations and mental health: Middle age and older men and women from three European ethnic groups. *Research on Aging, 2,* 445–469.

Lazarus, R. S., & Folkman, S. (1948). *Stress, appraisal, and coping.* New York: Springer.

Leary, T. (1957). *Interpersonal diagnosis of personality: A functional theory and methodology for personality evaluation.* New York: Ronald Press.

Lieberman, M. A., & Glidewell, J. C. (Eds.). (1978). Helping processes [Special issue]. *American Journal of Community Psychology, 6*(5).

Lieberman, M. A., & Mullan, J. T. (1978). Does help help? The adaptive consequences of obtaining help from professionals and social networks. *American Journal of Community Psychology, 6,* 499–517.

Lieberman, M. A., Mullan, J. T., & Heller, K. (1990). *Social ties, social support, and recovery from bereavement.* Unpublished manuscript, University of California, San Francisco.

Lieberman, M. A., & Stilliger, C. (1990). *Impact of large group awareness training.* Unpublished manuscript, University of California, San Francisco.

Lieberman, M. A., & Tobin, S. S. (1983). *The experience of old age: Stress, coping and survival.* New York: Basic Books.

Lieberman, M. A., & Videka-Sherman, L. (1986). The impact of self-help groups on the mental health of widows and widowers. *American Journal of Orthopsychiatry, 56,* 435–449.

Lieberman, M. A., & Yalom, I. (in press). Brief group Psychotherapy for the spousally bereaved: A controlled study. *International Journal of Group Psychotherapy.*

Lindemann, E. (1944). Symptomatology and management of acute grief. *American Journal of Psychiatry, 101,* 141–148.

Menaghan, E. G., Pearlin, L. I., Lieberman, M. A., & Mullan, J. T. (1984). Life events, role conditions and adaptation: A panel study of social stress. In S. A. Mednick, M. Harway, & K. M. Finello (Eds.), *Handbook of longitudinal research: Vol. 2. Teenage and adult cohorts* (pp. 255–272). New York: Praeger Scientific.

Mortimer, J. T., Finch, M. D., & Kumka, D. (1982). Persistence and change in development: The multidimensional self-concept. Vol. 4 of P. B. Baltes & O. G. Brim, Jr. (Eds.), *Life-span development and behavior* (pp. 264–308). New York: Academic Press.

Mullan, J. (1981). *Parental distress and marital happiness: The transitions to the empty nest.* Unpublished doctoral dissertation, University of Chicago.

earlin, L. I., & Lieberman, M. A. (1978). Social sources of emotional distress. In Roberta Simmons (Ed.), *Research in community and mental health: Vol. 1* (pp. 217–248). Greenwich, CT: Jai Press.

Pearlin, L. I., Lieberman, M. A., Menaghan, M. A., & Mullan, J. T. (1981). The stress process. *Journal of Health and Social Behavior, 22,* 337–356.

Rosenberg, M. (1965). *Society and the adolescent self-image.* Princeton, NJ: Princeton University Press.

Rosenberg, M. (1979). *Conceiving the self.* New York: Basic Books.

Rosner, A. (1968). *Stress and the maintenance of self-concept in the aged.* Unpublished doctoral dissertation, University of Chicago.

Wortman, C., & Silver, R. (1987). Coping with irrevocable loss. In G. R. Vanden Bos & K. Bryant (Eds.), *Cataclysms, crises, and catastrophes: Psychology in action* (pp. 185–235). Washington, DC: American Psychological Association.

Yalom, I., & Lieberman, M. A. (in press). Spousal bereavement and heightened existential awareness. *Psychiatry.*

7

Late-Life Adaptation in the Aftermath of Extreme Stress

Boaz Kahana

The study of extreme stress has emerged in recent years as an identified and distinct area for scientific inquiry. Initially research has centered around war trauma, focusing on shared symptomatology among war veterans who have participated in the Vietnam War, the Korean War, World War I, and World War II (Figley, 1985). Studies of Holocaust survivors revealed evidence of a similar posttraumatic reaction (Kahana, Harel, & Kahana, 1988). The Society for Traumatic Stress Studies was established in 1985 and began to attract research dealing with diverse trauma. It was soon recognized that common elements exist in the reactions of victims and survivors to war, natural disasters, rape, family violence, hostages, violent crimes, and occupational hazards (police, fire fighters, and personnel working with trauma survivors). The focus of this chapter is on extreme stress and the elderly, an area that could also be illuminated by the insights of traumatic stress studies. Conversely, gerontological insight may provide useful and new perspectives for consideration of processes and sequelae of extreme trauma. A major goal of this chapter is the identification of a range of issues that can be subsumed under the study of extreme stress and aging. A brief review of research findings is provided in each of the areas considered. Illustrations are also given from several research projects conducted by the author to test directly research questions framed in conceptual approaches of traumatic stress research that focuses on the elderly.

Although the study of extreme stress has many common elements with general stress research, it also provides some important departures and opportunities for clarification. There is a great deal of controversy in the general stress research literature regarding the degree to which stress is a stimulus external to a person (e.g., a stressor) or a response that reflects the inability of a person to deal successfully with problems. There is also debate about what constitutes a stressor, with individual differences in appraisal playing a central role in defining stressful life events. Although adverse health and psychosocial sequelae of life stresses have been demonstrated, research has also focused on coping, social supports, and other resistance resources that have been shown to have moderated the adverse effects of stress.

In contrast to the preceding, in the field of traumatic stress there is far less doubt about the nature and definition of stressors. Trauma and catastrophe are terms used to distinguish extreme stress from stress in general. Such extreme stresses are set apart by their overwhelming, life-threatening, unpredictable quality that cannot be mastered through normal problem-solving efforts. They represent life-threatening events and external traumas of such overwhelming magnitude that individual differences in appraisal appear to be of limited relevance. In fact, a unifying theme of traumatic stress studies has been that diverse traumatic stresses have shown long-term consequences, labeled "post-traumatic stress disorder" (PTSD), and have been found to affect victims of war trauma as well as those subjected to traumatic stressors in civilian life.

How applicable are conceptions developed in general stress research for the comprehension, analysis, and understanding of the impact of these most extremely stressful conditions? Some authors dealing with natural disasters, prisoner-of-war camps, concentration camps, and combat have preferred not to use the term *stress* and have chosen the term *extreme situations* (Hass & Drabek, 1970). Torrance (1965) reviews and discusses natural disasters as part of this larger category and defines them as follows: "Situations involving threats of, or experiences of an interruption of normally effective procedures for reducing certain tensions together with a drastic increase in tension to the point of causing death or major personal and social readjustment may be called extreme situations" (Torrance, 1965, p. 1). Bettelheim and Torrance also prefer to use the terms *extreme conditions* and *extreme stress.* Torrance (1965) suggests that distinct elements in extreme situations are the lack of conventional social structure, the loss of an anchor in reality, and the lack of the ability to predict or anticipate outcomes. This formulation also has its basis in the description of concentration camp conditions (Bettelheim, 1960), where individuals had little or no ability to anticipate and predict outcomes on a day-to-day basis. Extended situations of physical degradation, deprivation, lack of food, extreme cold, and prolonged isolation were elements that characterized life in concentration camps and in some prisoner-of-war camps. An additional important factor was the absence of conventional social structure. As a consequence, in concentration camps and other extreme conditions, conventional modes of behavior were rarely applicable. In addition, duration of extreme stress and its course were, in most instances, unpredictable. Consequently, individuals in such situations were called on to respond to conditions for which they were unprepared. At the same time, individuals in those circumstances were aware that failure to respond adequately resulted in severe consequences for them, including the constant threat of death. Authors, reviewing studies of inmate behavior in concentration camps (Chodoff, 1970) identified several converging themes. These included excessive anxiety, emotional distance, helplessness, depression, psychosomatic illnesses, continued preoccupation with the experience, and a variety of other physical and psychiatric disorders (Kahana, Kahana, Harel, & Rosner, 1988).

PTSD

Symptoms of PTSD appear consistently in the aftermath of war and other man-made disasters in which the identity and self-concept of the victim are attacked. It is less consistently observed subsequent to natural disasters.

Although the exact symptoms associated with PTSD may vary, and diagnostic classifications have undergone an evolution to reflect recent research findings in this area, several of the following major categories of disturbance are included (American Psychiatric Association, 1987):

1. Reexperiencing the traumatic event through flashbacks, dreams, and repetitive or intrusive thoughts.

2. Avoidance responses that include numbing to feelings, denial, withdrawal from the environment, and avoidance of activities that are reminiscent of traumatic event.
3. Hypervigilence, anxiety, and excitability.
4. Impairment in concentration and sleep disturbances.
5. Increase in symptoms when exposed to events reminiscent of the trauma.

The terms *victim* and *survivor* are alternatively used in the literature to describe persons who have experienced extreme stress or trauma. The term victim reflects the suffering and adverse consequences of the trauma, whereas the term survivor embodies endurance and ability to rebound and remain intact even in the face of adversity. Thus, although the early focus of research on traumatic stress has been on common *adverse* sequelae of trauma, our own research (Kahana, Harel, & Kahana, 1989) has underscored the important duality referred to earlier by documenting both deficits in mental health and proactive responses aimed at healing and integration of the later-life sequelae of earlier trauma (White, 1974). The critical adaptive tasks during extreme trauma are those of self-preservation. In the aftermath of trauma, adaptive tasks change to limit adverse effects of intrusive and disturbing memories of the trauma. Long-term effects of past trauma have also been postulated to cause exaggerated responses and to increase the effects of present stresses (Lomrantz, 1990).

CLASSIFICATION OF TYPES OF EXTREME STRESS RELEVANT TO AGING

In considering extreme stress and aging, two major categories of research must be distinguished. The first category deals with later-life sequelae of traumatic experiences earlier in life, whereas the second category refers to responses to extreme stress that are encountered in later life.

Stressors of Old Age

It should be noted that the distinction between stressors studied in the field of general stress research and those considered by researchers in the area of extreme stress often become blurred when stresses endured by the elderly are considered. Thus it has been acknowledged (Pearlin & Lieberman, 1979) that the stress of loss is a major characteristic of older adults. Furthermore, losses in later life often entail bereavement and health decline and may share much in common with stressors generally studied in the framework of extreme stress research. During periods of increasing frailty physical illness may present extremely stressful life experiences (Moos & Schaefer, 1979). Anticipation of extreme stress and particularly of one's own mortality is a seldom noted but universally salient form of extreme stress confronting the elderly. For many older persons the fear and reality of entering a nursing home, with concomitant disruption of one's normal environmental social structure also present situations that contain some elements of extreme stress (Kahana, Kahana, & Young, 1987).

Aging and Stress—Processes

Does old age require specific considerations in understanding long-range sequelae of earlier stress? Why would the elderly be differentially affected by extreme stress? Possible reasons may be fruitfully considered in the framework of special jeopardy suggested by researchers on stressors among social minorities. Smith (1985) reviews five hypotheses related to social groups that may be of specific risk in terms of the stress paradigm. These include the victimization hypothesis, the differential exposure hypothesis, the vulnerability hypothesis, the additive burden hypothesis, and the chronic burden hypothesis. The definitions of these hypotheses are as follows:

1. The victimization hypothesis refers to the selective nature of certain forms of trauma in preying on older persons.
2. The differential exposure hypothesis implies that older persons have an increased risk of exposure to certain forms of extreme stress (e.g., bereavement).
3. The vulnerability hypothesis suggests that stresses with a limited impact on younger persons have a more adverse effect on older people who may have reduced adaptive capacities (Rosow, 1967).
4. The additive burden hypothesis suggests that the elderly have accumulated many more stressful life experiences than their younger counterparts and that additional negative life events place them at a greater risk for negative outcomes.

5. The chronic burden hypothesis refers to the long-term effect of extreme stress that was experienced earlier in life.

The victimization hypothesis and the differential exposure hypothesis may be most readily applicable to extreme stressors of later life that involve victimization such as elder abuse or criminal victimization of inner-city elderly. The vulnerability hypothesis may be most readily applied to those elderly who confront natural disasters late in life. In terms of later life sequelae of earlier trauma resulting from life crises or war or other trauma experienced earlier in life, the additive burden hypothesis and the chronic burden hypothesis have particular salience.

There are several reasons for anticipating that the precarious equilibrium obtained by survivors of trauma may be disrupted in later life. Older people are particularly vulnerable to stress because of diminished social and environmental resources (Kahana, Kahana, & Kinney, 1990). There may be a diminished sense of control in later life resulting in depressive responses to stressors such as war related events (Hobfoll, Lomrantz, Eyal, Bridges, & Tzemach, 1989). Increased incidence of chronic illnesses and a growing awareness of nearness to death may add to the vulnerability of older adults as reminders of the severe assault on the self caused by earlier trauma. In some instances such as survivors of the Holocaust, even encounters with the health system may be frightening; survivors may view illness as a death sentence because those who were physically compromised in the concentration camps were routinely exterminated. Illness may also stimulate identification of the survivors with the world of death (Lifton, 1988). The elderly are also frequently confronted with reminders of their own mortality through the illness and death of friends and family, which are among the most commonly experienced life events among the elderly.

The elderly often confront life events that present threats to their own well-being or that of their loved ones. Thus, physical health symptoms of the self or spouse or sensory loss are likely to result in anticipation of negative outcomes. Such stresses may flood the older adult with memories of traumatic experiences and may remind them that the environment presents major threats to them. Increasing frailty of old age may require older persons to redefine their self-concept in recognition of their diminished control of the environment.

A key concept for considering the impact of extreme stress on later life is that of vulnerability. Vulnerability may be defined as the increased probability of negative outcomes in response to trauma (Kahana et al., 1990). Such increased vulnerability may be a function of increased exposure to trauma and diminished resources. Exposure to trauma is increasingly likely with age in terms of health-related cataclysmic events (such as strokes and amputations), and in terms of elder abuse (which occurs in the form of family violence directed at the aged). Diminished resources that render older adults particularly vulnerable may be in the form of external resources such as low income, substandard housing, or lack of a social support system (Kahana et al., 1990), or in the form of diminished coping resources or coping strategies (Clark, 1982; Elwell & Maltbie-Crannel, 1981).

DEVELOPMENTAL VIEWS

Responses to trauma may be viewed in the context of life-course development and may be influenced by life stages in which they occur (Elder & Clipp, 1988; Laufer, 1988). Thus it may be argued that trauma in childhood or adolescence will have a more pervasive effect on personality than trauma experienced during the adult years. Trauma during the early stages of development is also likely to influence modes of coping with future stresses. Trauma experienced in later life, conversely, could have particularly profound effects on psychosocial well-being because of the "environmental docility" situation in which older individuals are found (Lawton & Nahemow, 1973).

In addition to the differential impact of trauma that occurs during different periods in the life cycle, a developmental perspective is also useful for considering the impact of trauma on human development. Victims and survivors of trauma are likely to experience alterations in their social as well as psychological development. Such alterations may be due to an altered milieu such as a lack of work or job opportunities, or absence of an extended family (Kahn & Lewis, 1988). They may also be due to the adverse effects of trauma, or the inability to form social relationships (maintain intimacy) or to sustain generativity in those individuals who suffer from PTSD. In addition, the impact of trauma may alter psychological development of processes such as the life review in older adults (Butler, 1968). Thus, traumatized individuals may hypothetically have adverse emotional reactions to reviewing life experiences that may not have a traumatic impact on less traumatized persons. In considering posttraumatic coping of survivors, use of a life-cycle developmental perspective permits us to focus on positive concerns of survivorship. Life-cycle theorists anchored in ego psychology such as Erikson (1950) have called attention to the gradual accumulation or personal coping resources over a person's life. Successful resolution of each developmental crisis may lead to coping resources that may be mobilized in dealing with subsequent crises. Thus, it may be anticipated that successful resolutions of developmental crises lead to a sense of efficacy and ego integrity in later life (Moos & Billings, 1982).

METHODOLOGICAL CHALLENGES IN THE STUDY OF EXTREME STRESS IN LATER LIFE

In terms of methodological approaches, the study of extreme stress in later life is at a very early stage of development, with relevant work being largely descriptive in nature and often based on samples of convenience. Conceptually, however, the study of extreme stress presents some noteworthy advantages in relation to research in other areas of stress. In most cases extreme stress is an undeniable external reality in which appraisal or other aspects of coping play a more limited role than in the study of lesser stresses. Similarly, when dealing with milder stresses, individual differences represent a powerful factor in consideration of outcome. There is, in contrast, extreme trauma of diverse origins that results in a standard clinical syndrome of PTSD. The direction of causality is also clear in the study of extreme stress because the negative well-being outcomes are unlikely to create extreme or traumatic stress (i.e., a "recursive model"). In contrast, nonrecursive models are far more plausible in other areas of stress research. Thus, depression within the individual would obviously not result in his or her exposure to earthquakes or war trauma, whereas depression could just as well be the cause of an individual's divorce or a consequence of divorce.

Inferences of causal sequelae present a lesser problem in the study of extreme stress than in the general field of stress research, whereas consideration of the later-life impact of stress endured early in life presents different conceptual and methodological challenges. It is difficult to disentangle the relative impact of major trauma of natural or man-made disasters from the impact of the attendant stressors at reentry into normal society and normalized life situations. Furthermore, the researcher must consider a layering of trauma experienced by an older person who had been exposed to prior extreme stress. Such cases include the range of life crises experienced by the person (e.g., loss of parents or prolonged unemployment); the special trauma of war (e.g., combat duty or incarceration); the reentry experience (stigma of disabilities, disrupted family relationships, or reestablishment in an occupation); and, finally, recent life events (e.g., widowhood). In studying responses to extreme stress endured early in life among older adults, the researcher is also hampered by the problem of recall. Thus, there is evidence that events such as the "Day of Infamy" for Pearl Harbor survivors or concentration camps for Holocaust survivors are recalled in great and vivid detail with intrusive memories of trauma indelibly etched in the psyche of survivors (Kahana et al., 1989). There may be less accuracy in recall of stresses during the reentry period, however, such as the early days of immigrant life among Holocaust survivors.

EMPIRICAL PERSPECTIVES ON THE SEQUELAE OF EXTREME STRESS ON LATER LIFE

The later-life sequelae of extreme stress have been considered in two separate investigations by the author and his associates, focusing on two different populations of elderly persons. Findings that illustrate the conceptual issues outlined earlier will be briefly reviewed here to underscore commonalities as well as differences in late-life sequelae of extreme stress that affect a broad spectrum of older persons.

The major research project that has been recently compiled by the author and his associates (Kahana, Harel, & Kahana, 1988) considered physical and mental health and adaptation to aging among older adults who had survived the Nazi Holocaust. One hundred fifty Holocaust survivors who had immigrated to the United States and 150 Holocaust survivors who had immigrated to Israel were studied and compared with two groups of Jewish older persons who had, respectively, migrated from Europe to the United States and to Israel during the years immediately preceding the Holocaust. In a second study focusing on the later-life sequelae of wartime trauma, older U.S.

veterans who had been survivors of the Day of Infamy attack on Pearl Harbor (December 7, 1941) were studied (Wilson, Harel, & Kahana, 1989). The two studies differ in populations, research objectives, and research methods, but they share some important features. Conceptualization in each case reflected interest in the late-life sequelae of trauma experiences earlier in life, and consideration of social and personal resources that mediate the impact of trauma on later-life well-being.

The focus of studies of extreme stress, both in earlier and later life, has been on adverse somatic and psychological sequelae, particularly as exemplified by the symptomatology of PTSD. Studies have frequently focused on clinical populations such as those individuals who seek counseling or referral for psychiatric care. Seldom does research in this field also deal with social functioning and adaptation of survivors that reflect healing and integration. Few studies include nonpatient, community-based samples. Control or comparison groups have also been infrequently used. Furthermore, the earlier studies did not use standardized clinical research instruments but depended instead on global evaluations based on clinical psychiatric examinations (Kahana et al., 1988).

In our research focusing on both elderly survivors of the Holocaust and Pearl Harbor survivors, we interviewed nonclinical populations. We also considered indicators of wellness and integration along with adverse sequelae of trauma. Potential buffers of traumatic events in terms of social resources and individual coping resources were also considered. Finally, there was a beginning effort to address specifically the later-life experience of older adults who had endured traumatic events earlier in life.

Study of Elderly Survivors of Pearl Harbor

The study of elderly survivors of Pearl Harbor (Wilson et al., 1989) depicted the type and degree of psychological reactions left by traumatic experiences endured during the young adulthood stage of this group. In addition, it sought to explain correlates of later-life psychological well-being, in terms of degree of trauma experienced, social supports, coping strategies, and coping resources exhibited by survivors. There was no control or comparison group in this study. The sample ranged in age from 62 to 85 years with a mean age of 65 years.

Most were enlisted men (93%) with 72% having served in the navy and 18% in the army.

Measures of psychological sequelae of trauma include symptoms of PTSD and responses to the Bradburn (1969) Affect Balance Scale. Aspects of later-life coping resources and strategies included locus of control, altruism, and self-disclosure. Several other indexes were similar to those noted earlier in research of elderly Holocaust survivors.

In terms of exposure to stress, veterans who were survivors of Pearl Harbor reported high levels of combat exposure including being fired on, seeing comrades killed, and experiencing life and death situations. Forty-five years after the occurrence of this trauma 65% of veterans still experienced intrusive memories of the trauma, which represents a major criterion of PTSD. Survivor guilt was reported in 42% of the respondents with avoidance and hyperarousal reported by about one third of the sample. It is also noteworthy that one third of the veterans had difficulties expressing feelings about their traumatic experiences. When respondents were asked to compare symptoms that they experienced immediately subsequent to the war with later-life symptoms, there appeared to be some decline of symptomatology over time. The greatest decline occurred in the category of "intrusive imagery" and survivor guilt, whereas hyperarousal and avoidance diminished far less. The findings also reveal that combat exposure correlated strongly and significantly with PTSD ($r = .48$, $p < .01$). Negative evaluations of military service also correlated with PTSD ($r = .20$, $p < .05$) but more modestly. In terms of coping resources, those with external locus of control reported significantly greater symptomatology ($r = .32$, $p < .01$). Combat stress was also significantly correlated with negative affect ($r = .28$, $p < .05$) as was the receipt of medical care on discharge ($r = .28$, $p < .05$). In terms of coping resources, external locus of control was a significant correlate of negative affect ($r = .28$, $p < .05$).

Results of regression analysis confirmed the bivariate findings and suggested that both level of wartime stress and coping resources (the latter reflected in internal locus of control) were significant predictors of later-life well-being. Self-disclosure also emerged as a significant predictor of positive affective states. The data suggest that the ability to share experiences with others along with an internal locus of control may reflect an orientation that facilitates positive adaptation subsequent to the trauma (Wilson et al., 1989).

Study of Elderly Holocaust Survivors

A major goal of this research study (Kahana et al., 1988) was to determine whether a community sample of older adults who had experienced extreme trauma early in life differed significantly in well-being and mental health from a comparison group. A strength of this investigation is that, in addition to collecting data on 150 Holocaust survivors living in the United States and 150 survivors living in Israel, data were also collected on comparison samples of 150 adults in each of these two respective countries. The two comparison groups consisted of European refugees who left Europe for the United States and for Israel within 5 years before World War II. Respondents were thus matched on ethnic and cultural backgrounds and also on immigrant status. The Israel sample was included for the purpose of studying the potential inferences of cultural milieu on survivors as well as the possible effects of the sustained stress of living in a war-torn zone of the Middle East, surrounded by frequent threats to life and loss of family members and friends during five major wars since 1948.

Structured interviews with survivor and comparison groups covered such areas as reported physical health (Older American Resource Study [OARS] Subscale), mental health indices (Symptom Checklist–90 [SCL-90]), Morale (Lawton Morale Scale), and social functioning. In addition, coping strategies, family relations, and world outlook were investigated along with survivors' traumatic wartime experiences, including details of incarceration in camps and ghettos. The mean age of survivors was 63 years. The comparison group was slightly older. Seventy-one percent of the survivors are married to other survivors. Survivors maintain very traditional marriages with only 8% currently or previously divorced (3% currently divorced and 5% remarried from divorce). Religious affiliation is very strong and very traditional among survivors despite their Holocaust experiences. Fifty-seven percent reported conservative synagogue affiliation, and an additional 23% still report orthodox affiliation, with only 12% reform and 8% unaffiliated. Thus, an overwhelming 80% of survivors find meaning in traditional religious affiliation despite their Holocaust experiences and despite the frequently voiced question, "Where was God to save us?"

Results

Findings are first presented in terms of differences between survivors and comparisons in physical health, and regarding psychological dis-

tress. Next survivors and comparisons are compared on social functioning. Finally, findings are presented regarding factors that indicate
the relations between extreme stress early in life, and positive or
negative affect in later life.

In terms of physical health and pathology, results from this study
are consistent in certain ways with earlier investigations. Survivors
report more physical symptoms than our control group but only for
certain types of physical illnesses. Significantly greater proportions of
survivors reported symptoms that could be psychogenic in nature.
Thus, ulcers were reported by 20% of the survivors versus 4% of the
comparison group, and abdominal bloating was reported by 18% of
the survivors and by only 10% of the comparison group. Conversely,
no significant differences emerged between survivors and comparisons on such disorders as cancer, Parkinson's disease, and arthritis.
Regarding psychological symptomatology, there is clear evidence that
their traumatic experiences had an enduring effect on the survivors.
Thus, in response to the question, "How often do you think of your
Holocaust experiences?" 61% of the survivors said they did so either
daily or several times a week, and 75% thought of their experiences
at least once a week. Thus, survivors experience persistent and intrusive memories of traumatic events even 40 years or more after their
experiences.

In terms of psychological distress, survivors' SCL-90 primary
symptom dimension profiles were all significantly elevated relative to
both our comparison group and the standardized norms. It should be
noted, however, that most survivors obtained low scores on the
SCL-90 scales (i.e., a score of 1 or 2). In terms of morale, respondents' scores on the Lawton Morale Scale indicated several striking
differences between the survivor and control groups on 7 of the 17
items (feel lonely a lot; have a lot to be sad about; get upset easily; feel
life is difficult most of the time; afraid of many things; get mad more
than I used to; sometimes worry so much that I could not sleep at
night). On the more optimistic side, however, there were no significant differences between survivors and comparisons on 10 of the 17
items.

Results regarding social functioning present a noteworthy contrast
to physical health and psychological well-being outcomes relative to
the comparison sample. Although the survivors have significantly less
education, their income was significantly greater than that of the
comparison group. Survivors also had superior job histories and were

more apt to be gainfully employed. Survivors also demonstrated significantly greater residential stability and lower divorce rates. Finally, survivors experienced significantly greater feelings of responsibility toward their community. This was demonstrated through involvement in grass-roots organizations and the variety of volunteer roles that they undertook.

In integrating the findings of greater psychological distress among survivors, we may consider their responses as normal reactions to a very abnormal environment and series of events earlier in their lives. They are also reflective of posttraumatic stress reactions in the aftermath of traumatic life events (Figley, 1985). The findings regarding survivors' social functioning serve as testimony to an amazing resilience or hardiness (Kobasa, Maddi, & Kahn, 1982) reflected in the ability to cope with the adaptive tasks of life even after experiencing great adversity.

Regarding the influence of the Holocaust trauma on coping with the problems of getting older, less than half (45%) stated that the Holocaust made it more difficult for them to cope with aging; 29% said it made no difference; and, interestingly, 26% said it made it easier for them to cope with aging (i.e., "once you survive the Holocaust, you can survive anything"). The data indicate that most survivors see themselves as different from those who have not experienced the Holocaust. When categorizing these differences, it appears that many survivors view themselves as negatively affected (46% of those who said they were different), whereas almost as many reported strengths and positive features (34%). On examining more carefully those (34%) who reported positive sequelae after the Holocaust, three primary patterns emerged.

One group (27%) reflects greater idealism and concern for others (illustrated by statements regarding more humane, more empathetic, and more compassionate views toward others). The second group (36%) portrays the theme of greater appreciation of life ("I appreciate life more"; "I appreciate the U.S.A."; "I appreciate everything I have"). The third and largest group (46%) reports with pride the sources of strength that they found within themselves. Their strength encompassed physical stamina, strength of character, and better coping and resourcefulness.

The following four factors were significantly associated with greater positive affect among survivors:

1. Sharing wartime Holocaust experiences with family and friends correlated significantly with positive affect ($r = .37, p < .001$).
2. Having an altruistic orientation toward the world was significantly associated with positive affect ($r = .35, p < .001$).
3. Having an internal locus of control was significantly associated with positive affect ($r = .31, p < .001$).
4. Having a spouse who is also a survivor was modestly but very significantly related to positive affect ($r = .21, p < .001$).

The pervasive nature of efforts to cope with extreme stress during the later stages of adult development is illustrated in some unanticipated findings about differences in late-life stresses within the family as seen through some life events reported by survivors and the comparison group. Overall there were no significant differences in the total life-events scores of survivors and the comparison group. Consideration of specific clusters of events revealed noteworthy differences, however. Thus, among the survivors, there were significantly more life events involving illness of self and of spouse compared with the control group. At the same time, there were significantly fewer family problems reported by survivors. Survivors had fewer marital problems, and they were less likely to be divorced or separated. Survivors also had fewer problems with their adult children, and there was less divorce among their children. The data present compelling evidence about strong family ties and cohesiveness as adaptive responses among survivors who suffered dramatic losses of significant family members during the Holocaust.

Qualitative analysis of our data corroborates these observations. One survivor describes meeting his prospective wife immediately after the Holocaust as he went back to search for survivors and family in his hometown. He found one woman survivor, whom he befriended and subsequently proposed marriage. She had a problem with the proposal, however, because of her obligation to care for her frail father. The survivor had lost his father in the Holocaust, though, and wanted to care for the woman's father and view him as a father to both of them.

Other Man-Made and Naturally Caused Trauma

The effect of traumatic events on younger versus older people as well as the long-term effects of trauma on individuals as they age may be raised with the following additional groups: survivors of natural disasters (hurricanes, tornadoes, or floods); police and fire fighters, medical personnel working with trauma cases; hostages; survivors of criminal violence; and survivors of child abuse, incest, and rape. The literature is sparse regarding gerontological issues relevant to these traumata, with the exception of natural disasters.

Several studies are reported on older adults who were survivors of floods and other natural disasters. Results show that these events do adversely affect both the physical health and the mental health of those exposed to this stress. Furthermore, these effects have peaks at different points, with physical health peaks within the first year, functional impairments (i.e., performing day-to-day activities) peaking immediately after the event, and psychological symptoms portraying periodic fluctuation and being cyclical in nature (Phifer, Kaniasty, & Norris, 1988).

According to Friedsam's (1960) data on natural disasters, older people are likely to account for 2 to 3 times as many direct fatalities as would be expected from their percentages in an impact population. Injury and indirect casualty effects also appear to be higher among older persons in these disaster situations (Friedsam, 1960). Data from newer studies, however, do not portray more negative physical or mental health effects on the elderly as compared with younger age groups (Huerta & Horton, 1978; Kilijanek & Drabek, 1979). It should be noted, however, that Friedsam's study reports casualties, whereas the latter two studies are based on self-reports of survivors of a tornado and a flood.

CONCLUSION

Using this view, it may be useful for researchers on posttraumatic stresses to consider the survivor's mastery of prior experienced trauma as a coping resource that enhances a sense of competence. This in turn may lead to a perception of potential stressors as less threatening. Survivors may thus use reality-oriented coping (Haan, 1977) as a framework involving purpose, choice, flexibility, and adherence to logic. Indeed, there appears to be evidence that survivors cope in this competent manner to define problem situations—especially those that do not involve threats to health or survival. Thus, it appears that a review of post traumatic coping of survivors affords us a major opportunity for consideration of differential effects of stress in enhancing versus undermining the efficacy of coping. Indeed, extreme stress may selectively do both. Hence, the survivors may be condemned to doing battle with ghosts of the trauma, rehearsing in nightmares, and confronting them time and again in the face of minor illnesses or difficult situations. At the same time, the survivor may portray both ego strength and competence on the job or in navigating through bureaucracies that render the average person helpless and incompetent.

There has been an emerging literature providing conceptualizations appropriate to understand the impact of war trauma on adult development. The works of such investigators as Lifton (1988); Krystal, Giller, and Cicchetti (1986); and Laufer (1988) all converge to suggest that once a person is subjected to extreme stress, the trauma becomes embedded in the personality and stimulates further interactive relationships between memories of the trauma and subsequent changes in adult development. The fundamental problem in living through extreme trauma is that the personality and self-system of survivors will continue to be particularly grounded in the traumatic milieu. Yet after the war, people must return to function in conventional society. Various theorists have suggested alternative conceptualizations to explain this dissonant situation. Thus, concepts of serial self (Laufer, 1988) and doubling (Lifton, 1988) have been proposed to account for this conflict. In our own data, confirmation for these two distinct levels of being emerged. The traumatized self is reflected in our findings regarding psychological symptoms among survivors as compared with controls. At the same time, our data also reveal that survivors function remarkably well in the world of achievement and social contributions. This affirms the remarkable adaptive capacity of humankind even in the face of extreme trauma. For gerontologists, it is particularly salient to know that adaptability and achievement among traumatized adults persists well into later life.

Both survivors of the Holocaust and U.S. veterans of World War II who survived Pearl Harbor have experienced trauma of different kinds. Survivors of the Holocaust experienced victimization of the most inhuman kind, with almost no opportunity for control, in a surrealistic world of humiliation and torture. Veterans, conversely, were active warriors and victors representing their country. They were exposed to threats, combat stress, and life-threatening conflicts that began with being victims of the surprise attack on Pearl Harbor.

After the war, Holocaust survivors faced yet another trauma of displacement from their countries of origin and the need to adapt to a new environment as immigrants. In contrast, U.S. veterans were lauded as heroes by their country but still faced multiple problems of reentry into normal peacetime society. Yet, despite these differences, there were noteworthy similarities in long-term sequelae of extreme trauma among the two groups. Even 45 years subsequent to the critical traumatic events, these older survivors provided extremely vivid and detailed accounts of the Day of Infamy or their Holocaust experiences. This underscores the later-life reality of their trauma that was experienced much earlier in life.

Memories of trauma continue to intrude into the lives of these older adults, thereby testifying to the long-term duration of PTSD symptoms subsequent to war stress. At the same time, these data underscore the remarkable resiliency among long-term survivors of extreme stress (Shanan, 1989) and the important role of such coping resources as self-disclosure and internal locus of control in contributing to their psychosocial well-being subsequent to the trauma.

REFERENCES

American Psychiatric Association. (1987). *Diagnostic and statistical manual of mental disorders* (3rd ed., rev.). Washington, DC: Author.

Bettelheim, B. (1960). *The informed heart.* New York: Free Press.

Bradburn, N. M. (1969). *The structure of psychological well-being.* Chicago: Aldine.

Butler, R. N. (1968). The life review: An interpretation of reminiscence in the aged. In B. L. Neugarten (Ed.), *Middle age and aging* (pp. 486–496). Chicago: University of Chicago Press.

Chodoff, P. (1970). Psychological response to concentration camp survival. In H. Abram (Ed.), *Psychological aspects of stress* (pp. 44–61). Springfield, IL: Charles C Thomas.

Clark, A. W. (1982). Personal and social resources as correlates of coping behavior among the aged. *Psychological Reports, 31,* 577–578.

Elder, G. H., & Clipp, E. C. (1988). Combat experience, comradeship and psychological health. In J. P. Wilson, Z. Harel, & B. Kahana (Eds.), *Human adaptation to extreme stress: From the Holocaust to Vietnam* (pp. 131–156). New York: Plenum Press.

Elwell, F., & Maltbie-Crannel, A.D. (1981). The impact of role loss upon coping resources and life satisfaction of the elderly. *Journal of Gerontology, 36,* 223–232.

Erikson, E. (1950). *Childhood and Society.* New York: Norton.

Figley, C. R. (Ed.). (1985). *Trauma and its wake: The study and treatment of post-traumatic stress disorder.* New York: Brunner/Mazel.

Friedsam, H. J. (1960). Older persons as disaster casualties. *Journal of Health and Human Behavior, 1,* 269–273.

Haan, N. (1977). *Coping and defending: Processes of self-environment organization.* New York: Academic Press.

Hass, J. E., & Drabek, T. E. (1970). Community disaster and system stress: A sociological perspective. In J. E. McGrath (Ed.), *Social and psychological factors in stress* (pp. 264–286). New York: Holt, Rinehart and Winston.

Hobfoll, S., Lomrantz, J., Eyal, N., Bridges, A., & Tzemach, M. (1989). Pulse of a nation: Depressive mood reactions of Israelis to the Israel-Lebanon war. *Journal of Personality and Social Psychology, 56,* 1002–1012.

Huerta, F., & Horton, R. (1978). Coping behavior of elderly flood victims. *The Gerontologist, 18,* 541–546.

Kahana, B., Harel, Z., & Kahana, E. (1988). Predictors of psychological well-being among survivors of the Holocaust. In J. Wilson, Z. Harel, & B. Kahana (Eds.), *Human adaptation to extreme stress* (pp. 171–192). New York: Plenum.

Kahana, B., Harel, Z., & Kahana, E. (1989). Clinical and gerontological issues facing survivors of the Nazi Holocaust. In P. Marcus & A. Rosenberg (Eds.), *Healing their wounds: Psychotherapy with Holocaust survivors and their families* (pp. 197–211). New York: Prager.

Kahana, E., Kahana, B., Harel, Z., & Rosner, T. (1988). Coping with extreme trauma. In J. Wilson, Z. Harel, & B. Kahana (Eds.), *Human adaptation to extreme stress: From the Holocaust to Vietnam* (pp. 55–79). New York: Plenum.

Kahana, E., Kahana, B., & Kinney, J. (1990). Coping among the vulnerable elders. In Z. Harel, P. Ehrlich, & R. Hubbard (Eds.), *The vulnerable aged: People, survivors and policies* (pp. 64–85). New York: Springer.

Kahana, E. F., Kahana, B., & Young, R. (1987). Strategies of coping and post-institutional outcomes. *Research on Aging, 9,* 182–199.

Kahn, M. D., & Lewis, K. G. (Eds.). (1988). *Siblings in therapy.* New York: Norton.

Kilijanek, T. S., & Drabek, T. E. (1979). Assessing long-term impacts of a natural disaster: A focus on the elderly. *The Gerontologist, 19,* 555–566.

Kobasa, S. C., Maddi, S. R., & Kahn, S. (1982). Hardiness and health: A prospective study. *Journey of Personality and Social Psychology, 42,* 168–177.

Krystal, J. H., Giller, E. L., & Cicchetti, D. V. (1986). Assessment of alexithymia in posttraumatic stress disorder and somatic illness: Introduction of a reliable measure. *Psychosomatic Medicine, 48,* 84–94.

Laufer, R. S. (1988). The serial self: War trauma, identity, and adult development. In J. Wilson, Z. Harel, & B. Kahana (Eds.), *Human adaptation to extreme stress: From the Holocaust to Vietnam* (pp. 33–53). New York: Plenum.

Lawton, M. P., & Nahemow, L. (1973). Ecology and the aging process. In C. Eisdorfer & M. P. Lawton (Eds.), *The psychology of adult development and aging* (pp. 619–674). Washington, DC: American Psychological Association.

Lifton, R. J. (1988). Understanding the traumatized self: Imagery, symbolization and transformation. In J. P. Wilson, Z. Harel, & B. Kahana (Eds.), *Human adaptation to extreme stress: From the Holocaust* (pp. 7–31). New York: Plenum.

Lomrantz, J. (1990). Long-term adaptation to traumatic stress in light of adult development and aging perspectives. In M. A. P. Stephens, J. H. Crowther, S. E. Hobfoll, & D. L. Tennenbaum (Eds.), *Stress and coping in later life families* (pp. 99–121). Washington, DC: Hemisphere.

Moos, R. H., & Billings, A. G. (1982). Conceptualizing and measuring coping resources and processes. In L. Goldberger & S. Breznitz (Eds.), *Handbook of stress: Theoretical and clinical aspects* (pp. 212–230). New York: Free Press.

Moos, R., & Schaefer, J. (1979). The crisis of physical illness: An overview and conceptual approach. In R. Moos (Ed.), *Coping with physical illness: Vol. 2. New perspectives* (pp. 3–25). New York: Plenum.

Pearlin, L. I., & Lieberman, M. A. (1979). Social services for emotional distress. In R. Simmons (Ed.), *Research in community and mental health: Vol. 1* (pp. 217–248). Greenwich, CT: Jai Press.

Phifer, J. F., Kaniasty, K. Z., & Norris, F. H. (1988). The impact of natural disaster on the health of older adults: A multiwave prospective study. *Journal of Health and Social Behavior, 29,* 65–78.

Rosow, I. (1967). *Social integration of the aged.* New York: Free Press.

Shanan, J. (1989). Surviving the survivors: Late personality development of Jewish Holocaust survivors. *International Journal of Mental Health, 17*(4), 42–71.

Smith, J. R. (1985). Rap groups and group therapy for Vietnam veterans. In S. M. Sonnenberg, A. S. Blank, & J. A. Talbott (Eds.), *The trauma of war: Stress and recovery in Vietnam veterans* (pp. 125–163). Washington, DC: American Psychiatric Press.

Torrance, E. P. (1965). *Constructive behavior: Stress, personality, and mental health.* Belmont, CA: Wadsworth.

White, R. W. (1974). Strategies of adaptation: An attempt at systematic description. In Coelho, G. V., Hamburg, D. A., & Adams, J. E. (Eds.), *Coping and adaptation* (pp. 47–68). New York: Basic Books.

Wilson, J., Harel, Z., & Kahana, B. (1989). The Day of Infamy: The legacy of Pearl Harbor. In J. Wilson (Ed.), *Trauma, transformation, and healing* (pp. 129–156). New York: Brunner/Mazel.

8

Stress, Health, and
the Minority Aged

Richard W. Hubbard

The purpose of this chapter is to review some of the critical issues regarding clinical and research perspectives on the relationship between stress and health in minority elderly populations. First, it should be noted that there is a relative paucity of research data available on this and many other topics related to the minority elderly. Research problems for this particular area range from subject recruitment difficulties to the lack of culturally appropriate measures for stress and subjective well-being. In terms of stress-health relationships, measurement problems abound. To understand the complexity of the issues involved it is necessary to examine and challenge some of the assumptions many researchers and clinicians seem to make about ethnicity, stress, and health.

Essentially this chapter makes the following arguments:

1. Stress measures that are developed with and for predominantly white populations are inappropriate for use with minority populations.

2. When stressful event measures are used, they may overestimate the amount of stress the older minority group member is actually

Portions of the research and writing time of the author were supported by a grant from the Retirement Research Foundation, Chicago, Illinois.

experiencing. Such measures emphasize trauma and stressful events and will typically cast the minority elder as disadvantaged in comparison with white counterparts. This may in turn lead researchers to infer a higher level of subjectively experienced stress in the minority aged on the basis of these differences. The fact of the matter may be that minority elderly are more experienced and resourceful in coping with such stressors and therefore less affected by them.

3. The types of events that minority elderly find stressful may have a direct impact on their health status; however, we have yet to identify fully what these events are and therefore cannot describe their true impact on physical health.

4. Once stressful situations such as low income are adapted to and managed, they may no longer be stressful, unless the stress-management system employed (e.g., budgeting, problem-solving skills) breaks down because of an additional stressor such as changes in public-assistance eligibility requirements or substantial increases in costs of food and housing.

5. If our approach to stress and physical health measurement is based on the demographics related to illness and certain major life events, then minority elderly will be found to be at a severe disadvantage. If we use measures that rely on self-reports of the subjective experience of stress or physical health, however, such group differences may decline or disappear.

FACTORS INFLUENCING STRESS SCORES IN MINORITY SUBJECTS

Stress has proved to be a multifaceted and somewhat elusive construct which has generated an enormous volume of research. When the variable of ethnicity is added to an already complex construct, several errors and confounding variables may arise. For example, it is widely accepted that positive events such as marriage, buying a new home, moving, and other life-style changes are potentially stressful. If minority elderly are denied opportunities for some of the positive transitions of aging, such as moving to a home more adequate for retirement years, traveling on extended vacations, and so on, they may in fact score lower on stress event scales that include such items. Of course, the fact may be that the lack of opportunity for such events may be more stressful than their occurrence. This suggests that questions related to recent experiences with discrimination, or feeling as though one has been denied something by virtue of race, may be important domains for stress measures used in minority research.

Subject selectivity must also be considered in this regard, because morbidity and mortality rates are significantly greater for minority elderly. If we use age 70 or higher as a cut-off point for subjects we are effectively excluding many minority elderly who may have been victimized by the greater stress they experienced in their early or late 60s.

Stress has been routinely conceptualized as a complex biopsychosocial event. Each of these spheres may be components of the stressor itself (e.g., physical illness, loss of social status, or grief) or components of the reaction to stress on the part of the individual (e.g., some forms of gastric illness, social withdrawal, or anxiety and depression). Further complicating measurement and theory in the area are the various types of stress: trauma versus hassles, acute episodes or events versus chronic long-term conditions that individuals encounter. The word "stress," much like the word "depression," has become a common descriptor for several conditions that people encounter. This poses a problem for researchers who may be defining stress in a very different way from their subjects.

Obviously, such issues loom even larger when the study involves people of different cultural heritage. For example, consider the researcher who wishes to study stress related to transportation difficulties. In a middle-class, white, suburban community, he or she may find that transportation stress is quite strongly related to factors such as mechanical problems with one's car, driving in traffic jams, and poor weather conditions. Further, the researcher may discover that this group of subjects views taking a bus as an additional stressor, rather than as a coping measure for a transportation problem. Public transportation for these subjects may be viewed as an additional inconvenience and in many cases as an unknown. Now consider the same investigation in a low-income, inner-city, community of minority older persons. For such groups, the lack of a car may not be viewed as a stressor as long as public transportation is available and affordable. In other words, for one group public transportation may be in and of itself a stressor, whereas for another it is an effective coping measure for the management of transportation needs.

This rather simplistic example strikes at an important perspective on stress as a concept applied to the minority elderly; high levels of stress may occur when the management system applied to cope or handle a given problem fails. Thus, a low-income minority elderly person may only experience transportation-related stress when a public transportation route is changed or when they can no longer afford the fees. If we apply a white, suburban, stress-events model to such groups, by asking them if they have an automobile or when it last broke down, we may *infer* a level of stress that is simply not present. Table 8.1 offers examples of a life-conditions, stress-management, stressors model that may explain why older minority individuals who are disadvantaged and victimized by certain events or conditions may not report experiencing correspondingly high levels of stress. In this model stress occurs when the management system used to cope with the event or condition breaks down. Thus, aging plays a factor not in increasing the number of stressful life conditions but in threatening well-developed management systems for coping with lifelong conditions.

Although this model does not fully explain the stress-health relationship for minority elderly, it does suggest that minority elders may be more resourceful copers than some have suspected. The contribu-

TABLE 8.1 Life-Conditions, Stress-Management, Stressors Model

Life conditions	Stress management	Stressors
Lack of reliable automobile	Use of public transportation	Route changes, weather delays, fare increases
Poor access to health care services	Folk medicine, home remedies, in-home care from family, uses of public health services	Illness requiring surgery, chronic disease; loss of family members; changes in location or eligibility criteria of public health agencies
Low income	Budgeting, bartering, intergenerational supporting, cost sharing	Increased health care, housing, food costs
High rates of criminal victimization	Family, neighborhood, home-security plans	Increased fear, anxiety, costs, and social isolation when security breaks down

tions of stress that old age may provide needs to be analyzed in terms of its impact on fairly extensive systems of coping aimed at managing a variety of living circumstances.

STRESS, HEALTH, AND THE MINORITY ELDERLY

The increased morbidity and mortality rates among minority elderly, particularly African Americans, Hispanics, and Native Americans have been well documented (Jackson, 1989; Markides & Mindel, 1987). What is less well understood is the relative contributions of several variables to this significant and alarming trend. If, for example, these rates are the tragic consequence of the lifelong experience of discriminatory practices involving denial of health care services and abject poverty, then future generations (with their gains in civil rights and socioeconomic levels) should show morbidity and mortality rates that more closely approximate those of their white counterparts.

The group differences in morbidity and mortality do not appear for the first time in the later years of life. In fact, they are life-span phenomena, beginning with tragic differences in infant mortality. In other words, what appears to be happening is that minority persons encounter a shortened life expectancy at birth that continues to be true in old age (Ferraro, 1987). The only exception to this trend is a crossover effect in old-old age when black elderly actually gain in life expectancy in comparison with whites. From this perspective, the argument could be made that we ought to consider old age to begin 5 or 10 years sooner for minority elderly and apply various service eligibility criteria accordingly.

The double-jeopardy hypothesis stating that the discrimination and negative social attitudes and practices toward the aged combine with institutional and social racism to place minority elderly in double jeopardy regarding health and life satisfaction has gained some support from research (Dowd & Bengtson, 1978; Markides & Mindel, 1987). Clearly, inadequate health care brought about by poverty, poor access to services, and the lack of cultural sensitivity in health education and health promotion programs, for example, will all contribute to increased morbidity and mortality in minority elderly populations.

Conversely, the double-jeopardy hypothesis and other research as well (see, e.g., Biegel & Farkas, 1990; Shimkin, Shimkin, & Frate, 1978) suggest that lifelong discrimination and subculture membership may lead toward the development of protective resource management and coping particularly within families. Thus, as Eysenck's (1982) stress-inoculation hypothesis suggests that prior experience with stress contributes to the aged person's ability to cope with future stressors. Age leveling has been suggested as a process in which the problems that all aged face actually reduce the differences in disadvantages seen in younger ethnic groups.

One of the more striking aspects of the morbidity and mortality rates of minority elderly (and for white elderly as well) is the degree of life-style involvement with disease states such as hypertension, lung cancer, liver disease, and cardiovascular dysfunction that afflict them. High-risk illness behaviors such as smoking, overeating, and heavy alcohol consumption have all been shown to be stress related (e.g., Riley, Matarazzo, & Baum, 1987), and in fact stress-management techniques are one of the commoner components in programs designed to alter such behaviors. These links underscore the importance of considering stress-health relationships because it tends to put responsibility for health in old age squarely in the hands of the older person more than any medical or technical advance or specialty.

The critical questions for considerations then become: Are the minority elderly under greater stress than their white counterparts? If so, is this difference age related or a life-span process that may have more critical outcomes in old age? Consider the following scenarios that develop from this research perspective:

1. If increased levels of stress are lifelong patterns for minority elderly then in many cases we may be encountering more experienced, resourceful coping behaviors on the part of this group in comparison with their less experienced white counterparts.

2. If older minority persons have had to extend their coping resources more fully than whites throughout the life-span, then we may identify groups of minority aged who encounter the stressors of old age with a depleted or overextended set of coping responses.

In other words two models begin to form. One casts the minority elderly as better prepared for coping with old age than their white counterparts by virtue of greater previous experience with stress, change, and trauma. The other suggests that the addition of new or greater levels of stress for the minority elderly may come at a time when their resources are already depleted, thereby rendering them more vulnerable to the impacts of stress on physical health.

Either model must account for the following, well-established facts:

1. At present, minority elderly have greater morbidity and mortality rates than their white counterparts. This does not appear to be a consequence of aging, rather it is a life-span phenomenon.

2. Although several biological and social explanations for this trend may be put forth, one of the more well-studied mitigating factors for morbidity appears to be stress. Correspondingly, a body of evidence linking coping style to health is continuing to grow.

3. These observations lead to the hypothesis that minority elderly may be experiencing greater levels of stress than whites, and that this may in turn at least partially explain the well-documented differences in health between these groups.

Stress and the Minority Elderly

Research regarding stress and the minority elderly is by no means uniform in its results. Some researchers have found significant differences for instance between black and white elderly on measures of stress and well-being, with the black elderly having greater stress and less well-being; others have found little or no difference (see, e.g., Chatters, 1988; Jackson, 1988). The most important coping variables associated with older blacks and Hispanics appears to be family and church. This finding is particularly important because researchers have tended not to include church participation, nearness of the church to the home, home visits by clergy, and so on in examining the levels of support in minority elderly lives.

In a recent study conducted by this author, groups of alcoholic and nonalcoholic black elderly were studied across several variables including subjective levels of stress as measured by the Perceived Global Stress Measure (Cohen, Kamarack, & Mermelstein, 1983) and physical health conditions. All of the subjecs were low-income, inner-city elderly with one or more chronic illnesses. On face value such demographics suggesting poverty, chronic illness, and their associated stressors would lead us to hypothesize high levels of stress. Further strengthening this hypothesis is the fact that half of the subjects included in the study were diagnosed as alcoholics. The results on the 14-item stress measure that has a score range from a low of 0 to a high of 56 indicated that both the alcoholic (mean score of 25) nonalcoholic (mean score of 24.83) groups had low to moderate levels of perceived stress. It is also important to note that there were no significant differences in perceived stress between the alcoholic and nonalcoholic groups, even though the alcoholics tended to have greater physical illness and functional limitations. The measure did correlate positively with number of falls in the last 2 months, suggesting that acute incidents may increase the perceived level of stress when they interrupt an ongoing stress-management coping strategy.

The items on the Perceived Stress Scale measure focus on failure to cope, asking the frequency with which an individual has encountered feelings of lack of control, anger, nervousness, ability to cope, and feeling overwhelmed. It does not focus on specific events. Thus, what we appeared to encounter in this pilot study with a small sample of subjects is the very pattern referred to earlier: Individuals experiencing a significant number of stressful conditions do not report high perceived levels of stress, perhaps because they were managing the conditions successfully.

What seems to emerge from research data in this area is that although the double-jeopardy hypothesis receives support from demographics regarding the physical and psychosocial conditions of the minority elderly, it does not receive strong support from their subjective reports of stress or well-being.

Reformulation of Research Questions

If we accept the convincing data regarding increased stressful events and health problems among the minority elderly and note the equivocal findings regarding the subjective levels of stress and perceived well being in these groups, we are faced with reformulating our research questions. It is well documented that there are cultural variations in the way health and illness are defined and experienced within different subgroups (Spector, 1979), and it may well be that the same is true for stress. Further complicating our understanding of the process is the fact that different cohorts of elderly will bring with them different sets of experiences and attitudes regarding stress and health.

How do minority elderly define stress? The following hypotheses need to be tested:

1. Cultural differences in the way in which interpersonal conflict is interpreted as stressful exist. Given the higher value placed on interpersonal communications and relationships in some Hispanic groups, for example, we might find that stress in this sphere is rated more negatively than economic or physical stressors.

2. Locus of control issues will interact with levels of perceived stress in minority elderly. Again, we can borrow from a growing literature (see, e.g., Jackson, 1989) to determine the degree to which feeling personally in control of one's life will influence subjective experience of stress.

3. If morbidity in the minority elderly is linked to health behaviors regarding alcohol use, nutrition, and exercise, then we would expect the incidence of alcohol problems, obesity, and lack of exercise to be higher in these groups. If alcohol and overeating are being used as stress-coping mechanisms, such findings would emphasize the importance of culturally sensitive health and wellness programs for such groups.

4. The changes in income, physical well-being, and family that have been well documented in the later years of life may occur on a much steeper gradient for middle- and upper-class individuals of any race than for persons at lower socioeconomic levels. In other words the relative changes in health, finances, and social support experienced by the elderly may be mitigated by the degree to which these variables were present in the middle years of life. Thus, old age may in fact be a much more stressful period of life for upper- and middle-class individuals than for the predominantly minority lower socioeconomic classes.

CONCLUSION

Psychosocial stress is a hypothetical construct, and as such it will be redefined and better articulated by research. Considerations of stress and health in the minority elderly will contribute to this process as they begin to examine the ways in which minority elderly define, experience, and cope with stress. At present it seems clear that minority elderly may be different from their white counterparts across all three of these dimensions.

Obviously, how stress is defined and measured will directly influence the pattern of results obtained. As discussed in this chapter, a model that predicts significantly lower and higher levels of stress can both be generated and defended by the currently available data. It may be time to "begin at the beginning" and explore how stress is defined by the minority elderly rather than to superimpose existing models developed primarily with whites on to a variety of other cultures.

REFERENCES

Biegel, D. C., & Farkas, K. J. (1990). The impact of neighborhoods and ethnicity on black and white vulnerable elderly. In Z. Harel, P. Ehrlich, & R. Hubbard (Eds.), *The vulnerable aged: People, services and policies* (pp. 116–136). New York: Springer.

Chatters, L. M. (1988). Subjective well-being among older black adults: Past trends and current perspectives. In J. Jackson (Ed.), *The black American elderly: Research on physical and psychosocial health* (pp. 237–258). New York: Springer.

Cohen, S., Kamarack, T., & Mermelstein, R. (1983). A global measure of perceived stress. *Journal of Health and Social Behavior, 24*, 385–396.

Dowd, J. J., & Bengtson, V. L. (1978). Aging in minority populations: An examination of the double jeopardy hypothesis. *Journal of Gerontology, 33*(3), 427–436.

Eysenck, H. J. (1982). Stress, disease and personality: The inoculation effect. In C. L. Cooper (Ed.), *Stress research: Issues for the 1980s* (pp. 213–234). New York: Wiley & Sons.

Ferraro, K. F. (1987). Double jeopardy to health for black older adults? *Journal of Gerontology, 42*, 528–533.

Jackson, J. (1989). Race, ethnicity, and psychological theory and research. *Journal of Gerontology, 44*, 1–2.

Jackson, J. (Ed.). (1988). *The black American elderly: Research on physical and psychosocial health.* New York: Springer.

Markides, K. S., & Mindel, C. H. (1987). *Aging and ethnicity.* Beverly Hills: Sage.

Riley, M. W., Matarazzo, J. D., & Baum, A. (1987). *Perspectives in behavioral medicine: The aging dimension.* Hillsdale, NJ: Erlbaum.

Shimkin, D. B., Shimkin, E. M., & Frate, D. A. (1978). *The extended family in black societies.* The Hague, The Netherlands: Mouton.

Spector, E. E. (1979). *Cultural diversity in health and illness.* Norwalk, CT: Appleton-Century-Crofts.

PART III
Reducing Adverse Effects of Stress: Practice and Intervention

This section focuses on the diversity of approaches to dealing with stress and offers new insights into alternatives to more costly medical management of the late consequences of stressful situations. It covers a broad spectrum of approaches toward therapeutic intervention for stressed older persons. In several of the chapters, these approaches include interventions designed to reduce or eliminate physical and psychological responses to stress. Kennedy discusses the biological factors associated with stress and symptomatology that stress may cause in the absence of known diseases that ordinarily produce these symptoms. Conversely, he also describes the relationship of depression to disease. He provides a basis for recognizing common symptom complexes for different problems. He discusses factors that affect therapeutic effectiveness of various agents, not only for simple depression, but also in anxiety states and PTSDs.

Baldwin surveys the environment as a moderator of stress. The chapter describes two projects involving a multiplicity of factors that cause increased or decreased strain on personnel. These contain modules for training staff to cope with stress and understanding the cause of stress, a strategy that has resulted in an increased sensitivity to behavior. Through staff awareness of their own behavior-coping procedures, the stress of relocation and adjustment can be dealt with effectively. Baldwin also describes the physical phenomena associated with stress in these settings and iatrogenic responses to the relocated patients, particularly regarding staff attitudes and expectations.

Gatz discusses psychological interventions in the management of stress. She describes the concepts of primary prevention, secondary prevention, and remediation, depending on the timing in relation to the stressful situation. She develops a model of coping that involves interventions in situations leading to stress and tensions such as chronic strains and stressful life events. Gatz reviews the need for appropriate social resources and development of coping skills. Included also are interventions to minimize recurrence of stress. Her intervention strategies use the concepts of control, self-efficacy, and perceived confidence.

Walz and Brown focus on family-based, long-term care in dealing with stress. They provide a demographic basis for focusing on family-level caregiving. In their model, the formal health and social services have a secondary place and supplement the family caregivers. Walz and Brown build on a definition of family care that distinguishes it from community-based care, and they extensively review both positive and limiting features. The importance of family integrity is stressed. Walz and Brown discuss factors that impact on the family's responsibility for care in the current environment and potential difficulties placed on family caregivers in caring for an aged, dependent individual. They place consideration on the variation of stress thresholds among individuals as well as economic considerations in the family model and make recommendations for alternative systems of remuneration to support this level of activity.

9

Psychopharmacological Management of Stress in the Elderly

John S. Kennedy, M.D.

The term *stress*, is resistive to an operationalized definition. As applied to individuals, stress is understood to describe a response, an adaptive process "to environmental or internal demands that exceed an individual's capacities or resources" (Shader, Kennedy, & Greenblatt, 1987). From this perspective, stress responses of individuals are necessarily the result of the interaction of biological factors (genotypic-phenotypic characteristics); psychological factors (experience and style of interaction with the external world); as well as social factors (such as the availability or nonavailability of external resources). Also following from this perspective is the view that although stress itself is not a primary affective state (Shader et al., 1987), symptoms of stress may include many possible cognitive-affective phenomena such as fear, worry, or anxiety.

In the mental health sense, stress responses may be viewed as nonpathological when they are time limited and reality based, and result in mastery of coping skills and behaviors that permit conscious choice to avoid similar future experiences. Today few risk factors have been identified that specifically allow prospective differentiation of individuals who will develop pathological stress syndromes, such as some forms of the anxiety disorders, from those who will not. Anxiety disorders present as persistent fearlike affective responses defined by the presence of a specific clustering of mood, cognitive, physiological, and behavioral signs and symptoms (American Psychiatric Association, 1987).

BIOLOGICAL FACTORS ASSOCIATED WITH ANXIETY SYMPTOMS

In the elderly, physical disorders such as hypoxia and thyroid dysfunction are common. These and many other medical problems often initially manifest with predominantly psychological features. Medical conditions and the older person's social realities and consequent vulnerability to the effects of factors such as poverty and crime frequently interact adversely with age-associated increases in dependency. A clinical consequence of this is that separation of symptoms contributed by biomedical disorders, stress, adjustment disorders, fear, and anxiety disorders can at times prove very difficult (Shader et al., 1987). The medical differential diagnosis of anxiety symptoms is quite lengthy as is illustrated in Table 9.1. Many of the disorders listed in Table 9.1 are more commonly present with severe depression but as is true of primary depression in the aged, frequently anxiety symptoms may predominate.

One concomitant of aging is the accumulation of a burden of chronic medical disorders so that the likelihood of the aged individual having a medical disorder is higher than in the younger population. For this reason, no elderly individual should be seen in a psychotherapy context without having had a recent comprehensive medical evaluation. This is particularly appropriate for the older individual who presents for the first time with symptoms that may benefit from psychological therapy. The nonmedical clinician needs to recall that by the time the human achieves age 70 plus, very few individuals are unable to report significant life events that might readily explain their demonstrating psychological phenomena reflecting distress that is "understandable." The numbers of aged individuals, seen in psychotherapy in the community for "understandable problems" is unknown, but clinical impression suggests that it is common. It is still unfortunately common to encounter aged individuals who have expended significant amounts of scarce financial resources on inappropriate therapy offered in the absence of an adequate medical evalua-

TABLE 9.1 Partial List of Medical Conditions Associated with Anxiety-Like Symptoms

Endocrine-Metabolic-Nutritional
  Hypocalcemia or hypercalcemia
  Hypocortisolemia or hypercortisolemia
  Hypoglycemia or hyperglycemia
  Hypoparathyroidism or hyperparathyroidism
  Hypopituitaism or hyperpituitaism
  Hypothyroidism or hyperthyroidism[a]
  Hyponatremia
  Hypomagnesia
  Hypothermia
  Hyperkalemia
  Stress-induced antidiuretic hormone states
  Carcinoid syndrome
  Pheochromocytoma
  Insulinoma
  Porphyria
  Thiamine deficiency
  B-12 deficiency[a]
  Nicotinic acid deficiency
  Monosodium glutamate
  Ovarian dysfunction
  Testicular deficiency
Gastrointestinal
  Ulcer
  Diverticulitis[a]
  Ulcerative colitis
  Gastric dumping syndrome
  Irritable bowel syndrome[a]
  Pancreatitis
  Pancreatic carcinoma
Autoimmune
  Allergies
  Anaphylaxis
  Polyarteritis nodosa
  Rheumatoid arthritis
  Systemic lupus erythematosis
  Temporal arteritis[a]
Infectious
  Atypical viral pneumonia
  Brucellosis

(continued)

TABLE 9.1 (continued)

Malaria
Mononucleosis
Pneumonia
Scabies
Tuberculosis
Viral Hepatitis
Cardiovascular-Pulmonary[a]
    Anemia
    Angina pectoris
    Arrhythmias of any type
    Asthma
    Cerebral hypoxia and anoxia
    Chronic obstructive pulmonary disease
    Congestive heart failure
    Hyperventilation syndromes
    Hypertension
    Hyperdynamic beta-adrenergic states
    Mitral valve prolapse
    Myocardial infarction
    Pulmonary emboli
    Postprandial syncopal attacks
Neurological-Psychiatric
    All organic brain syndromes[a]
    Benign paroxysmal positional nystagmus
    Brain tumors
    Cerebrovascular disease
    Central nervous system infections
    Combined systemic disease
    Early Meniere's disease
    Epilepsy (Anencephalic partial complex, temporal lobe, ictal anxiety)
    Essential tremor[a]
    Major depression[a]
    Malingering
    Multiple sclerosis
    Myasthenia gravis
    Narcolepsy
    Pain states
    Parkinson's disease
    Personality disorders
    Polyneuritis
    Post-head injury

TABLE 9.1 (continued)

Schizophrenia
Sensory deficits (visual and auditory)
Sleep deprivation
Sleep disorders
Wilson's disease
Delirium
Medication-Associated
  Akathisia (neuroleptic-related)
  Aminophylline
  Amphetamines
  Atropine eyedrops
  Benzohexal
  Caffeine
  Clonidine
  Cocaine
  Diethyl propion hydrochloride
  Digitalis
  Ephedrine
  Epinephrine
  Fluoxetine
  Fluramine hydrochloride
  Guanethidine
  Hyoscine
  Hematropine
  Indomethacin
  Isoproterenol
  Levodopa
  Mecamylamine
  Methyldopa
  Methylphenidate
  Nicotine
  Norepinephrine
  Orphedrine
  Pentylenetetrazol
  Physostigmine
  Procyclidine
  Pseudoephedrine
  Reserpine
  Salicylates
  Sodium lactate
  Theophylline

(continued)

TABLE 9.1 (continued)

Tricyclic antidepressants
Yohimbine
Medication-Withdrawal–Associated
  Alcohol
  Benzodiazepines (especially short-acting)
  Barbiturates
  Clonidine
  Neuroleptics
  Opiates
  Tricyclic antidepressants

Note. Sources include Psychiatric Presentation of Medical Illness: Somatopsychic Disorders by
R.C.W. Hall, 1980, New York: Spectrum.
ªCommoner medical problems in the elderly.

tion. Some medical problems appear to be commoner in the elderly
and as a result necessitate consistent initial evaluation. These conditions are noted in Table 9.1.

In summary, the most important therapeutic principle that treatment should follow, not precede, characterization of the individual's
current state is a result of the reality that similar symptoms can reflect
different problems and often require very different treatments. Combined psychological and pharmacological therapy has an important
and valuable role in treatment of stress and related disorders, and can
particularly benefit the elderly person adjusting to the presence of
well-managed medical problems when the focus of combined therapy
is well formulated.

PHARMACOKINETIC AND
PHARMACODYNAMIC CONSIDERATIONS
IN THE ELDERLY

It is widely appreciated today that the elderly individual may show
different sensitivity to drug dosages appropriate for younger patients.
This is not to say that in all elderly individuals dosages necessary to
treat younger patients are inappropriate. It is clinically evident that as
in other domains, the elderly are heterogeneous. To account for the

evident differences in the response of many older adults to medication pharmacokinetic-pharmacodynamic studies in the elderly have been conducted, and findings relevant to some elderly individuals can be summarized. Medications that are lipophilic (enter easily into fat stores) such as diazepam are widely distributed within the body, and because in aging, particularly in women, the volume of distribution may increase, medications given in single dosages may be less persistently available at drug receptors and therefore may be less effective. Medications that are lipophilic may also accumulate if given frequently because the larger volume dispersal may take longer to be emptied, and therefore effects of such medications can be observed for longer than is expected in other age groups. Other age-related changes in the average characteristics of human physiology are also potentially significant including declining amounts of blood proteins (albumin) to which some medications attach. With medications that are readily attached to circulating proteins, small reductions in the amount of protein can cause substantial increases in the amount of medication circulating freely (unbound) in the blood and therefore increase the amount of medication available to attach to receptors at muscles and nerves. In such cases dosages of medications need to be lowered. The liver and kidneys are also of potential importance in how drugs are broken down. Changes in some enzyme systems in the liver (oxidative phase 1 system) can result in prolonged availability of medications such as diazepam, which is seen particularly in men. Pharmacokinetic-pharmacodynamic studies in the elderly further suggest that as a result of normal brain changes the number of receptors for some medications (such as nitrazepam) may decline, and thus dosing needs to be lowered (Greenblatt, Abernethy & Shader, 1986). For these reasons, "starting low, going slow and not hesitating to say no" are important rules of pharmacotherapy in the elderly. These rules must be clarified to include the reality, reflecting the heterogeneity of the elderly, that dosages that are ineffective should either be stopped or increased to effective amounts. Such decisions are made most often by evaluation of achieved benefit and considered against the presence and risk of side effects. The prescribing physician needs to reassess the patient frequently to enable optimal therapeutic dosing to be determined. Frequent clinical evaluation of patients is essential to good care. This expensive reality is in part a consequence of the very few reports of clinical trials of commonly prescribed psychotropic medications in the elderly population.

TREATMENT

Adjustment Disorders

It is unknown if pharmacological therapy results in any change in the natural history of adjustment disorders in the elderly. Perhaps reflecting the desire to reduce anguish and discomfort, medications have been consistently suggested to have a role, but this view is supported primarily by clinical wisdom alone. In instances in which medication use appears warranted, the choice most often involves selecting from within the available benzodiazepine class of compounds (Table 9.2). Certain benzodiazepine medications (oxazepam, lorazepam, and temazepam) may have a preferred role because of age-related changes in benzodiazepine pharmacokinetic profiles (Shader & Kennedy, 1989). Such therapy should be provided for symptoms such as sleep difficulties that are to some extent disabling and not simply uncomfortable. The regimen should be reviewed for need on a frequent basis, and an attempt to discontinue pharmacotherapy should be undertaken within a 3-month period.

TABLE 9.2 Benzodiazepines Currently Available in the United States

Generic name	Brand name	Indication
Alprazolam	Xanax	Anxiety
Chloriazepoxide	Librium	Anxiety
Clonazepam	Klonopin	Seizure disorders
Chlorazepate	Tranxene	Anxiety
Diazepam	Valium	Anxiety
Flurazepam	Dalmane	Insomnia
Halazepam	Paxipam	Anxiety
Lorazepam	Ativan	Anxiety
Midazolam	Versed	Intravenous sedation
Oxazepam	Serax	Anxiety
Prazepam	Centrax	Anxiety
Temazepam	Restoril	Insomnia
Triazolam	Halcion	Insomnia

Generalized Anxiety Disorders

For therapy of anxiety disorders such as generalized anxiety, in addition to the role of benzodiazepine, a trial of serotonergic neurotransmitter system modulating medication such as buspirone is warranted. Buspirone is the first available agent in the class of serotonin 5-HT$_{1A}$ receptor modulators; several other similar agents are currently being evaluated. Buspirone reportedly possesses only minimal ability to impair cognition, or muscle tone and motor coordination. It also has been marketed as lacking measurable abuse potential, abstinence syndrome, or physical dependence liability. In limited study to date it has similar pharmacokinetic characteristics in young and old. A recently reported study of buspirone in 605 elderly patients with anxiety resulting from a primary anxiety disorder or with anxiety in association with an affective state or personality disorder, oral dosages of 5 mg 3 times per day for 4 weeks produced improvement in 86% of patients rated by physicians' impression and in 81% of patients as self-reported by patients. Common reported side effects included dizziness (7.8%), stomach complaints (6.4%), and sleeplessness (4.5%). Nearly 20% of patients entered into the study discontinued therapy, 7% for reasons of side effects and 6% for reasons of insufficient efficacy (Robinson, Napoliello, & Schenk, 1988). Thus, in the elderly buspirone appears to be a relatively safe and effective treatment for primary anxiety disorders. If a clinical trial is attempted with buspirone the patient must be advised that 4 to 6 weeks may pass before any significant benefit manifests itself. Antidepressant or beta-adrenergic–blocking medications may also be of benefit for individuals with generalized anxiety disorder who fail to receive benefit from other approaches, but this remains controversial even in the literature on younger patients and has not been systematically studied in the elderly anxiety-disorder patient population.

PTSDs

The characteristic psychological presentation of the traumatically stressed older individual has been little described. Related to fear, it has been previously noted that behaviorally the older adult is often unable to make use of a fight-flight reaction set and may, under stress, instead show "freezing" behavior (Jarvik, 1980). Such behavior has been proposed to result from loss of speed (reaction time) or actual physical impairment that makes fight or flight impossible. Acute traumatic psychological stress has been reported to have devastating effects on some older individuals (Coakley & Woodford-Williams, 1979), but the incidence and outcome of trauma has not been systematically studied so it remains uncertain if the elderly are at greater risk for chronic posttraumatic stress than younger individuals. In the literature review for this chapter no citations or case reports on pharmacotherapy as an adjunct to supportive psychotherapy in this disorder were found specifically applied to the elderly.

Chronic, posttraumatic stress is likely a prevalent problem in the elderly and can be anticipated to increase particularly as the war-exposed generations in the United States continue to age. Traumatic stress is of course not limited to exposure to the horror of war and can present in association with natural disasters such as earthquakes, floods, or as a result of being a victim of crime or accidents. Few clinicians working in hospital orthopedics wards have not observed the fearful, dependent behavior of some elderly individuals who having fallen and broken a hip lay unattended for hours or days in their own home, in pain and with thoughts of death ever-present. Similarly, many nursing home staff have observed the mildly confused elderly male go on "guard duty" as night comes or the frightened Holocaust survivor seeking escape from "the camp." Symptoms of PTSD are evident in the patient's memory and often include the presence of intrusive ideations and nightmares. Emotional functions are also impacted with pervasive anxiety, irritability, anger, and depression among many possible manifestations. Cognitive functions are frequently affected so that attention span and concentration abilities are decreased. Typically sleep is disrupted, and the person frequently becomes socially withdrawn, develops difficulties in interpersonal relationships, and may become self-destructive.

Pharmacotherapy of PTSD can be seen to be an attempt to reduce the intensity of the patient's physiological and affective symptoms once the disorder has evolved and help is sought. Uncontrolled studies in young adults suggest that for some individuals pharmacotherapy is a useful adjunct to psychotherapy. In case reports almost every class of psychoactive medication has helped someone. Theoretically, based on assumptions concerning the neurochemical changes underlying symptoms formation such as an increased startle response in many victims, it has been argued that reduction of sympathetic arousal and anxiety employing agents such as the alpha-2 receptor-blocking medication clonidine or the beta-adrenergic receptor-blocking medications such as propranolol may be of particular utility (Kolb, Burris, & Griffiths, 1984). Unfortunately, the literature leaves unclear if such approaches are more or less likely to be of assistance than use of sedative-hypnotic, antidepressant, mood-stabilizing, or neuroleptic classes of agents (Friedman, 1988; Van der Kolk, 1987).

In summary, the pharmacotherapy of stress states in the elderly has not been subjected to systematic evaluation. Clinical impression suggests that subforms of stress, such as the anxiety disorders, are as likely to respond to medication as are similar states in younger patients. The major limitations clinically are the absence of recognition of such problems in the elderly cohort and the absence of systematic study of these problems. These limitations stem from an absence of general interest in the academic community in a group of problems that are believed to be quite common in the aged population. It is hoped that the next few years will bring a clarification of the operational description of stress problems such as traumatic stress in the elderly and thus provide a framework around which to test therapeutic intervention strategies.

REFERENCES

American Psychiatric Association. (1987). *Diagnostic and statistical manual of mental disorders* (3rd ed., rev.). Washington, DC: Author.

Coakley, D., & Woodford-Williams, E. (1979). Effects of burglary and vandalism on the health of old people. *Lancet, 2,* 1066–1067.

Friedman, M. J. (1988). Toward rational pharmacotherapy for posttraumatic stress disorder: An interim report. *American Journal of Psychiatry, 145,* 281–285.

Greenblatt, D. J., Abernethy, D. R., Shader, R. I. (1986). Pharmacokinetic aspects of drug therapy in the elderly. *Therapeutic Drug Monitoring, 8,* 249–255.

Hall, R. C. W. (Ed.). (1980). *Psychiatric presentation of medical illness: Somatopsychic disorders.* New York: Spectrum.

Jarvik, L. F. (1980). Anxiety and stress in the aged. In *Symposium* (pp. 29–43). Department of Psychiatry, University of Arizona. Nutley, NJ: Roche Laboratories.

Kolb, L. C., Burris, B. C., & Griffiths, S. (1984). Propanolol and clonidine in treatment of the chronic post-traumatic stress disorders of war. In

B. A. Van der Kolk (Ed.), *Post-traumatic stress disorder: Psychological and biological sequelae* (pp. 97–105). Washington, DC: American Psychiatric Press.

Robinson, D., Napoliello, M. J., & Schenk, J. (1988). The safety and usefulness of buspirone as an anxiolytic drug in elderly versus young patients. *Clinical Therapeutics, 10,* 740–746.

Shader, R. I., & Kennedy, J. S. (1989). Geriatric psychiatry: Biological treatments. In H. I. Kaplan & B. J. Sadock (Eds.), *Comprehensive textbook of psychiatry: Vol. 2* (5th ed., pp. 2037–2049). Baltimore, MD: Williams & Wilkins.

Shader, R. I., Kennedy, J. S., & Greenblatt, D. J. (1987). Treatment of anxiety in the elderly. In H. Y. Meltzer (Ed.), *Psychopharmacology: The third generation of progress* (pp. 1141–1147). New York: Raven.

Van der Kolk, B. A. (1987). The drug treatment of post-traumatic stress disorder. *Journal of Affective Disorders, 13,* 203–213.

10

Stress in the Elderly: Environments of Care

Beverly A. Baldwin

Institutionalization of the elderly has the potential for initiating and accelerating stress for the resident because of the nature of the institution itself, the number and type of health care workers interacting with the resident, and the multiple and interactive problems that an older adult may present when institutionalization is required. Clinical observations of the stressors encountered by elderly residents in nursing home settings during the last 4 years demonstrate the importance of the environment as a modifier of stress and the manner in which the nursing home setting, and its personnel and philosophy can significantly contribute to the escalation or diminishment of the stress and strain of being a patient.

STRESS OF PROVIDING CARE

A mental health training program was initiated in March 1986 as a demonstration pilot study. The purpose of the study was to ascertain the response of nursing home staff (both professional and nonprofessional) to training regarding the behavioral, emotional, and mental needs of residents in their care. A survey of the staff was conducted before developing the curriculum and content modules. Of the 50% (116) responding to interviews and questionnaires, almost 80% indicated a need to learn more about the stress of providing care and how to manage their own stress in the care setting. Fifteen modules were developed for the 116 staff members participating in the training program; three of the modules focused on stress and stress management for the staff. The program was conducted during a 1.5-year period. Each of the modules was presented 9 times each week to cover the number of staff members volunteering in this 184-bed intermediate-care nursing home. Modules were presented in small groups every other week. On the alternate weeks, a geropsychiatric clinical nurse specialist spent half of the time with the staff, reinforcing the content discussed in the seminars, and demonstrated effective management strategies for the staff. Sixty-seven of the staff members completed 12 of the 15 modules, and five of the staff members attended all the sessions. Pretest and posttest measures of attitudes toward the elderly and knowledge of behavioral problems were conducted, with no statistically significant differences in either measure before or after the training program. A follow-up interview with 20 of the 67 staff members completing the program indicated that even though they had difficulty retaining the didactic material presented in the seminar and reinforced clinically, they had learned and practiced stress-management strategies that they could individualize and implement in the practice setting. The pretest and posttest measures did not assess learning of the stress-management content. Staff indicated that an understanding of the causes of stress and specific modifiers of caregiving stress made them (a) more sensitive to the behavior being exhibited by the resident, (b) more aware of their own behavior and reasons behind their actions, (c) more aware of the stress activated by the residents' needs and staff-staff interactions influencing the care they provided on a daily basis, and (d) identify alternatives to the daily strain and stress encountered in the workplace, such as use of imagery, diaphragmatic breathing, and time-out. They also indicated that because stress management was included in the training program, its use and reinforcement with each other was legitimized. The need to understand the impact of personnel stress on residents cannot be overstated. Few systematic studies have examined the impact of caregiver stress on the resident and the reciprocal nature of stress between resident and staff member. Recent clinical studies and observations suggest this aspect of the nursing home environment is both more complicated and interactive than generally assumed (Burgio, Butler,

& Engel, 1988; Stevens & Baldwin, 1988; Tellis-Nayak and Tellis-Nayak, 1989).

STRESS OF RELOCATION AND ADJUSTMENT: A CASE STUDY

The State of Maryland, Department of Health and Mental Hygiene, Mental Hygiene Administration initiated a patient-transition management program in 1987 to provide follow-up for geropsychiatric patients relocated from state psychiatric facilities to private nursing homes in the state of Maryland. I was a member of the aftercare coordinator team, and the goal for this follow-up was to identify resident needs in the relocation process and evaluate the adjustment to the new setting and staff. Monthly visits were made to the nursing homes to evaluate the relocated residents and work with staff for the first 6 months after the transition. By March 1989, our team had followed 176 patients relocated into 41 nursing homes in central Maryland. The mean age was 69 years, with 64% (112) women and 36% (64) men. The initial recognition by the aftercare team was that the nursing home functions as a "behavior modifier," in that given the nature of the nursing home setting, conformity of residents is essential and reinforced. The staff expected rapid conformity by the transferred residents and had difficulty understanding the need for the resident to question or resist the routine of the home. For some of the homes, the tolerance level of the staff for nonconforming behavior of residents was high; for others, however, it was quite low and resulted in high stress levels for staff and relocated residents. This tolerance level varied among the nursing homes and resulted in a wide range of acceptance behavior by the staff. Some staff members had strict opinions regarding "appropriate behavior" to be exhibited by residents and the setting reinforced these narrow parameters for self-expression.

Also, the negative image of the nursing home, cited by some of the nursing staff, was reinforced by having psychiatric patients as residents. The attitudes of the staff regarding geropsychiatric patients, often without verification, resulted in an additional modifier imposed by the environment. Many staff were fearful or expressed anxiety about the resident's psychiatric illness even though more than 60% of the relocated patients had a diagnosis of dementia. These stereotypes and myths regarding the residents' psychiatric problems led to expectations of behavior. The nursing home policies and regulations regarding resident behavior reinforced these stereotypes of the staff, because little effort was noted to prepare staff for the needs and potential of the incoming patients. Much of the aftercare follow-up visit was spent in working with staff in this regard.

Family attitudes and response to the relocation played a part in how the nursing home "modified" the behavior of the resident. Most family members were positive to relocation, because being closer, geographically, facilitated visits for the resident. Some family members, however, felt the nursing home was not equipped to handle the mental health needs of their family member and expressed this to the staff in the nursing home. Individual work and consultation with family members was necessary to allay fears and anxieties regarding the nursing home staff's ability to handle the needs of the resident.

Adjustment Problems of Relocated Elders

Although numerous studies have documented the impact of relocation on elderly mortality, only recently have clinicians and researchers focused on the adjustment problems, both physiological and psychological, of the relocated or transferred (interinstitutional and intrainstitutional) elderly (Anthony, Proctor, Silverman, & Murphy, 1987; Elwell, 1986; Mirotznik & Ruskin, 1984; Stein, Linn, & Stein, 1985). Clusters of psychological adjustment problems were noted in the relocated residents including the exacerbation of delusions and hallucinations, wandering, behavioral excess (i.e., demanding cigarettes or overeating), restlessness, agitation, pacing, resistance to care (especially bathing, feeding, dressing, or toileting), verbal outbursts, mood swings, and sexual inappropriateness. The least tolerated behaviors included the sexual inappropriateness, aggressive or agitated behavior, and verbal abuse (especially racial slurs and curses directed toward the staff). As documented in institutional studies of cognitively impaired elders (Cohen-Mansfield, 1988), the more impaired the resident, the more agitated the behavior initially. Behaviors of residents that had been dormant in the psychiatric facility or handled effectively by psychiatric staff often become problematic for the nursing home staff. For most residents experiencing psychological adjustment problems immediately after relocation, however, these behaviors diminished or were effectively modified within 1 to 3 months after the transfer. Therefore, if nursing home staff could be instructed in management strategies, reinforced for effective approaches, and not overreact to the resident's behavior, the adjustment for the residents and the staff was overwhelmingly positive. Only 20 of the 176 residents had to be returned to the psychiatric facility during the first 2 years because of unmanageable behavior. One reason for the adjustment was the careful matching by psychiatric facility social work staff of patient's needs with nursing home resources and expectations. This was accomplished by the nursing home staff visiting the psychiatric facility to see the patient, indicating the type of patient their staff could manage effectively, and being able to call on facility staff (social workers and nursing staff) for assistance after the relocation. Additionally, the patient being considered for relocation could visit the nursing home being considered and decide if he or she liked the setting and could adjust to the change. Often family members accompanied the patient on the trial-day visit.

Adjustment problems stemming from physical care needs centered on six major areas: excessive weight gain or loss, skin breakdown, incontinence, urinary tract or respiratory tract infections, dehydration and electrolyte imbalance, and pneumonia. In some relocated patients, these physical problems could be predicted because of the patients' condition and the multiple and interactive chronic conditions. For some patients, however, these problems developed or were accelerated by the transition from a highly vigilant care setting to one in which the vigilance level was lower because of the level or number of staff members. Nursing home staff members found the more frail relocated resident stressful to manage; staff often assumed that because the resident was from a psychiatric facility, the physical care problems were secondary. The reverse was true for some of the transferred patients because it was indeed the physical care and functional disabilities that made them eligible for nursing home care and reimbursement via the state Medicaid system. For some of the residents experiencing physical problems, acute hospitalization was necessary; however, the frequency of these hospitalizations and acute physical care episodes decreased as the transition project progressed, and staff was more comfortable with the relocated residents and their needs. The aftercare follow-up provided an opportunity to reinforce the nursing care issues with the staff and to assist them in anticipating the needs of residents rather than focusing on crisis intervention or crisis reaction. As we enter the 4th year of the project, the number of acute care hospitalizations continues to decrease. Documentation of the stress experienced by the resident who has to be hospitalized is being carefully monitored to determine the effect on the health of the resident over time. Nursing home staff appears more comfortable with the physical care needs of the residents and is observed to actively anticipate resident needs immediately after transfer (i.e., encourage fluids, monitor eating and voiding patterns, and observe closely for signs of infection).

Iatrogenic Responses in Relocated Residents

Stressful events or episodes in the relocation process were observed to be directly related to the environmental milieu and staff reactions to individual residents. The environmental milieu and staff often did not recognize signs of homesickness in the residents, although many of the transferred patients had been institutionalized in a psychiatric facility for a long period (the range of institutionalization before transfer was 2 months to 40 years). For some of the relocated residents, the adjustment to the new environment, staff, and residents was difficult because they missed their friends, the staff of the psychiatric facility, or the physical unit where they had lived for several years. Some difficulty was experienced by nursing home staff in recognizing and responding to the homesick resident, because they did not understand why an elder would prefer the psychiatric setting over the nursing home setting. The environment was nonresponsive until it was pointed out that the residents would experience feelings of loss and remorse about leaving the familiarity and routine to which they were comfortable and accustomed.

Reverse stereotyping was noted in some nursing home staff. The assumption was made that because the residents were former psychiatric patients their physical care needs were not the highest priority. Therefore, some staff was observed to have unrealistic expectations of the residents regarding self-care or functional abilities, and this was particularly problematic in activities of daily living. The staff had some problem assessing the resident's abilities and independence, and often relied on the resident to determine what he or she could do alone, with minimal assistance. When it was pointed out that the resident needed assistance in understanding functional ability, the staff was more vigilant in this aspect of care.

Staff attitudes toward and expectations of resident's medication provided yet another example of iatrogenic responses. For some nursing staff, the realization that a resident was on a major tranquilizer indicated the resident must have "severe, bizarre, or difficult" behavior problems. It reinforced the myth regarding the underlying pathology of the resident's illness and required staff to receive instruction in the use of major and minor tranquilizers. It was important to reinforce the expected effects of the medications, and early signs and symptoms of side effects of the drugs with staff. Ministaff development programs were offered as part of the aftercare program to assist staff with this aspect of care, and nursing home in-service instructors were encouraged to include psychotropic medications in routine training programs in the nursing home.

A testing period was noted between residents and staff in some cases, particularly with residents with paranoid tendencies or who were suspicious of the setting or staff. The staff, in turn, appeared to be intimidated by those residents, and each would vie for control in the setting. The resident with these tendencies would test the limit setting of the staff and constantly try to gain control over the routine or the environment. Examples frequently occurring were limit setting about smoking cigarettes, bathing, toileting, or dressing. The staff had some difficulty realizing that the resident may need this initial time to "be in control" as part of the adjustment to a new environment and strangers. Ryden (1985) suggests the environment and boundaries of expectations can play an important part in promoting resident autonomy in the institutional setting. Flexibility and individualized routine setting were encouraged, especially during the early adjustment period, when the resident might feel more vulnerable to the new environment.

An unexpected iatrogenic response was noted in some situations in which the resident moved into the nursing home setting with little or no disruption in the nursing home routine. Rather than staff reacting to the resident as a "good" or "compliant" new admission, staff would forget the elder was new or was recently relocated. These residents tended to "blend in" with little or no response from the staff. On-site aftercare visits focused on the resident's need for recognition and planning for individual care, such as inclusion in social and recreational activities, orientation to the nursing home routine and to staff members, and careful evaluation of the resident's mood to determine the adjustment outcome. Concern was expressed to staff that these residents may become more withdrawn or depressed, with consequent physical care needs, which might not be observed if the resident did not receive careful and consistent observation and evaluation during the adjustment period.

Staff anxiety regarding the admission of a new resident from the psychiatric facilities varied from nursing home to nursing home, but the attitude of the home administration and nursing management were important in setting the tone for expectations of the resident. Staff in some of the nursing homes could not tolerate suspicious or paranoid residents, whereas this behavior was not problematic for staff in other homes. Assessment of the differences in attitudes and responses of staff in different settings is now under way, because this is an important component of psychosocial management in the institutional setting; the degree to which staff can be taught management strategies and attitudes can be changed has received little attention in the research literature. The need for careful evaluation of this component of care and staff's ability to respond to resident behaviors has been frequently noted (Burgio et al., 1988; Jackson et al., 1989; Kayser-Jones, 1984).

Staff Stress and Behavioral Needs of Residents

The relocation process and adjustment period provides an opportunity to observe the interrelationship of staff and resident stress over time. Observations to date indicate that process is both reciprocal and interactive, but the mechanisms by which it occurs requires further examination. In the nursing homes where staff appeared to have high tolerance for resident behavior, the "stress" level of the home was termed low by staff members. This was not found just in homes with low turnover rates and low percentages of part-time or temporary personnel. It varies from home to home based on both the staff's and administration's expectations of the transition program, the experience with similar residents, and the preparation the staff has for caring for the relocated resident. The attitudes of the administrative and nursing management personnel definitely impact the response of both professional and nonprofessional staff to resident behavior. The degree to which it impacts their response to the relocated residents is not clear, nor are the ways in which they can be altered or positively enhanced.

Environmental stressors noted in the nursing homes include a nonstimulating or nonsensory enhancing physical environment. This does not necessarily mean the lack of activity or recreational personnel, or depend on the size of the home. On the contrary, some of the smaller homes with less specialized personnel appear to have the most stimulating environments for residents. For these, the homelike environment and flexible routine accommodate the needs of individual residents for stimulation, whether in close physical proximity to staff and other residents or in activities that are integrated into the daily routine and that can facilitate resident abilities (i.e., afternoon outings for a snack or walk in a nearby park; or active volunteers, encouraging residents to participate in the activities of the day (cooking, table preparation, or simple housekeeping tasks).

Nursing staff frequently suggests that the long-term care environment is inherently a stressful setting, given the nature of the residents' problems and the limits of medical care possible. Many staff describe the nursing home setting as a form of hospice; however, little attention is given to the fact that, for many residents, the home is the last option before death. Because staff in the nursing home is not prepared like staff in the hospice setting to respond to resident needs and problems, the issues of death and dying are avoided, ignored, and often denied. There develops an unspoken conspiracy between staff and residents in which discussions of death and dying are avoided; cues are not recognized; and residents, staff, and family members do not openly acknowledge this aspect of the long-term care setting. This avoidance is stressful for both staff and residents, and may become an escalating problem as the resident becomes more debilitated and frail.

Consistent efforts are being made with the nursing homes accepting the relocated patients to provide for stress management for the residents by setting limits without becoming controlling and inflexible, encouraging control enhancement by the residents (i.e., promoting independence in activities of daily living, based on the resident's abilities; and allowing choices of food, routine, leisure, and recreational activities), and setting up consistent and congruent patterns of care for the individual elder. It appears that the more the resident knows what is expected from the relocation process and that he or she can rely on consistency of care, the less stressful the transfer is perceived. Immediate behavior modification strategies should be avoided, because the presenting behavior of the resident may not be the behavior exhibited once the adjustment period sets in. Allowing the resident to adjust "at his or her own rate" is reinforced in all the nursing home settings. There is great variability in the staff's tolerance of individualized behavior from the transferred residents.

POSITIVE ADJUSTMENT TO RELOCATION

The success of the transition program has been well substantiated in the number of patients who have adjusted well to the change in long-term care setting. Noted changes in behavior of residents and their family members attest to this outcome.

Residents who were not actively social in the psychiatric facility have been observed to interact more with other residents and staff, and participate in the activities (formal and informal) of the nursing home. The degree to which this positive aspect of the adjustment process is noted in individual residents varies, but, generally, the relocated residents have shown more interest in and involvement with activities in the nursing home environment.

Family involvement and visits have been one of the most positive outcomes of the program and resulted in reuniting some families and solidifying ties in others. Because the placement of the residents is planned so that they will be closer to the family or a family member, an increase in visits has been well documented for family members already maintaining contact with the geropsychiatric patient, and renewed ties and reestablished ties have been observed with family members who did not maintain contact with the resident while a patient was in the psychiatric setting. Family interest and involvement is a positive motivator for the nursing home staff to maintain active involvement with the resident, even when family-staff encounters are sometimes stressful (i.e., when family makes demands on the staff or express dislike about the resident's care). Staff contend that having the family active and caring about the resident is more important than the added stress this may create. Family members who have difficulty with the relocation are contacted individually, and aftercare follow-up is maintained throughout the period of adjustment for both resident and family. Many family members openly express satisfaction with the relocation and state this during visits with the resident. Staff-family conferences and telephone contacts are encouraged. Several of the nursing homes have family support groups, and the family members of the relocated residents have joined and find this type of support helpful in learning more about the nursing home, the elder's needs, and the role of the family in care of the resident. An increase in visits with families outside the nursing home has occurred in almost all cases in which the family has remained in close contact with the transferred elder.

CONCLUSION

The nursing home environment has been described as a stressful setting for elderly residents, given the nature of the setting and the staff-resident interactions that occur. Two projects, including training of staff and relocation of geropsychiatric patients, demonstrate the multiplicity of factors that contribute to the stress and ways in which the stressors for the residents and staff have been addressed. Further studies of stressful environments of care are needed to understand better the many etiologies of stress, effective management strategies for residents and staff, and evaluation of outcomes that differentiate positive from negative stress in long-term care environments.

REFERENCES

Anthony, K., Proctor, A. W., Silverman, A. M., & Murphy, E. (1987). Mood and behaviour problems following the relocation of elderly patients with mental illness. *Age and Ageing, 16*, 355–365.

Burgio, L. D., Butler, F., & Engel, B. T. (1988). Nurses' attitudes towards geriatric behavior problems in long-term care settings. *Clinical Gerontologist, 7*(3/4), 23–34.

Cohen-Mansfield, J. (1988). Agitated behavior and cognitive functioning in nursing home residents: Preliminary results. *Clinical Gerontologist, 7*(3/4), 11–22.

Elwell, F. (1986). The effect of single-patient transfers of institutional dependency. *The Gerontologist, 26*, 83–90.

Jackson, M. E., Drugovich, M. L., Fretwell, M. D., Spector, W. D., Sternberg, J., & Rosenstein, R. B. (1989). Prevalence and correlates of disruptive behavior in the nursing home. *Journal of Aging and Health, 1*, 349–369.

Kayser-Jones, J. S. (1984). Psychosocial care of nursing home residents. In B. Hall (Ed.), *Mental health and the elderly* (pp. 205–220). New York: Grune & Stratton.

Mirotznik, J., & Ruskin, A. (1984). Inter-institutional relocation and its effects on health. *The Gerontologist, 24,* 286–291.

Ryden, M. B. (1985). Environmental support for autonomy in the institutionalized elderly. *Research in Nursing and Health, 8,* 363–371.

Stein, S., Linn, M. W., & Stein, E. M. (1985). Patients' anticipation of stress in nursing home care. *The Gerontologist, 25,* 88–94.

Stevens, G. L., & Baldwin, B. A. (1988). Optimizing mental health in the nursing home setting. *Journal of Psychosocial Nursing and Mental Health Services, 26*(10), 27–31.

Tellis-Nayak, V., & Tellis-Nayak, M. (1989). Quality of care and the burden of two cultures: When the world of the nurses' aide enters the world of the nursing home. *The Gerontologist, 29,* 307–313.

11

Stress, Control, and Psychological Interventions

Margaret Gatz

Management of stress is a central element in the lives of older persons. The purpose of this chapter is to present ways in which psychological interventions can be used to help older individuals reduce or cope with stressful living situations. Conceptually, this chapter represents a merging of community psychology theories of intervention and social psychological theories of stress and coping, with an emphasis on the role of personal control. Consideration will also be given to how these models reflect the age of the target group, or whether age is of any relevance to effectiveness. In the past, many believed that older persons could not benefit from psychological interventions, a view that has largely been refuted (Gatz, Popkin, Pino, & VandenBos, 1985; Rodin, Cashman, & Desiderato, 1987).

The term *psychological interventions* encompasses planned interpersonal actions involving input from a trained professional that are intended to have a psychotherapeutic impact (Gatz et al., 1985). Using a community psychology perspective, interventions are traditionally described as primary prevention, secondary prevention, or remediation, depending on their timing (Caplan, 1964). Primary prevention occurs before a problem arises; thus, preventive interventions are directed at the causes of problems and distress. Secondary prevention occurs after a problem situation has been noted or a group has been identified as being at risk, but before serious difficulties have arisen. Remediation occurs after substantial problems or dysfunction have occurred; remedial interventions encompass diagnosis, therapy, and institutional care. The implication of a community approach is that most psychological interventions for reducing stress or helping people manage it constitute primary or secondary prevention, *not* remediation.

According to a community perspective, the target of preventive interventions is all older adults, anyone who might ever be stressed, not simply those already suffering from stress and not simply the even smaller subgroup of elders with diagnosable mental disorders. Indeed, it is important *not* to label those who are merely stressed as having a psychiatric diagnosis.

This stance can also be strategic if psychological services are provided under the rubric of stress management. Among people of all ages there is a preference not to view oneself as needing mental health services. The present cohort of older people have been accused of being particularly high on this form of reluctance (Lasoski, 1986). I am not convinced that this generalization is accurate (Gatz et al., 1985); nonetheless, if psychological intervention is presented as a course in coping with stress, it is far more palatable to many who could conceivably use the input but would avoid it under another name. Moreover, to the extent that older persons do avoid mental health professionals, at least one reason may be perceived irrelevance of the services being offered (Felton, 1982). Stress reduction, according to one elderly key informant at the Andrus Gerontology Center, is viewed as extremely pertinent to the perceived needs of older persons.

STRESS, COPING, AND HEALTH

To discuss the place of intervention in reducing stress, a model of stress is required. Many such models have been proposed, with many similar elements. In an admittedly arbitrary amalgamation, Figure 11.1 presents a model of stress that permits focusing on relevant elements of intervention (Lazarus & Folkman, 1984; Maddi, 1989; Pearlin, 1989).

The fundamental feature of these models is that some life event leads to poor health outcomes, mental and physical. It is inferred that

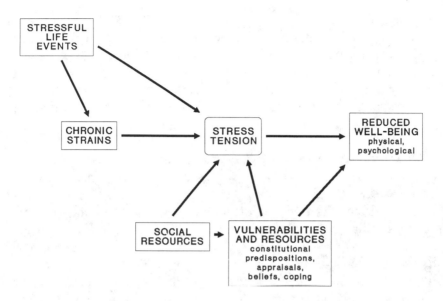

FIGURE 11.1 Amalgamated model of stress.

the event leads to stress which leads to the outcome. Mediators have often been added, especially personal resources, coping, and social support, which are encompassed here under vulnerabilities and social resources. The following discussion reviews each of these components of the model.

Stressful life experiences have been shown to be associated with increased vulnerability to physical illnesses and depression (Bloom, 1985; Holmes & Rahe, 1967). Pearlin (1989) in particular has elaborated the concept of the stressor. He divides stressors into life events and chronic strains.

A wide variety of dimensions has been used for classifying life events including positive versus negative, chosen versus imposed, major events versus daily hassles, and whether the stressfulness is determined objectively or whether salience is obtained subjectively. The most stressful life events tend to be those that are non-normative, unexpected, and negative (Gatz, Siegler, George, & Tyler, 1986; Hultsch & Plemons, 1979; Zautra, 1986).

Chronic strain can be described in terms of roles: having too many roles to fulfill, competition between roles, being placed in an unwanted role, and so forth (Pearlin, 1989). Often a life event leads to the chronic strain—for example, the event of death of a spouse leads to the chronic strain of widowhood including financial burdens, changes in social relationships, and other rearrangements. Furthermore, in thinking about intervention, it is also important that one person's life event can become the chronic strain of another family member; caregiving for an impaired parent is an obvious example.

The mediators represent factors that predict which individuals will suffer the greatest or the fewest negative outcomes after stressful events or because of stressful circumstances (Maddi, 1989). Mediators include constitutional predispositions, appraisals of the event and of one's ability to deal with it (Lazarus & Folkman, 1984), psychological resources (Lieberman, 1975), coping skills, and social support. Examples of constitutional predispositions would be family history of hypertension, tendency to have a migraine or colitis, and inborn temperament. Psychological resources that have been listed as leading to better adjustment to stressful life occurrences (with their opposites leading to less successful adjustment) include positive self-appraisals, sense of control, hope, sense of competence, and meaningfulness (Bloom, 1985; Lieberman, 1975). Coping skills have been categorized into three groups: changing the situation itself (behavior focused), changing the meaning of the situation (cognitive coping), and managing the stress (emotion focused) (Moos & Billings, 1982; Pearlin, 1989).

The final mediator is social resources. Following Dunkel-Schetter and Wortman (1981), Kahn and Antonucci (1981), and Thoits (1986), it can be said that there are three types of social support: tangible assistance, emotional support, and affirmation (i.e., validating feelings and providing information). As shown in Figure 11.1, mediators have direct as well as indirect effects on outcomes.

Outcomes include a wide range of physical health symptoms, anxiety, depression, and use of alcohol. It is important to note that life events do not inevitably cause mental health problems but could lead to maintenance of adjustment or to greater psychological well-being (Aldwin, chapter 4 of this book; Murrell, Norris, & Grote, 1987). There are individual differences; indeed, older adults may be more resilient than younger adults, possibly because of their accumulated past experiences in dealing with negative events (Norris & Murrell, 1988). Moreover, an ostensibly negative life event can result in positive as well as negative outcomes, such as personal growth and family solidarity that can result from one member's confronting a life-threatening disease.

Each step in the amalgamated model can be tied to concepts of control, efficacy, or autonomy. Is the person responsible for the occurrence of the stressful event, or has it occurred unexpectedly without planning? Elsewhere we (Gatz et al., 1986) have called this belief *locus-of-control event*. Does the person believe himself or herself responsible for managing the stressor? We (Gatz et al., 1986) have called this appraisal *locus-of-control handle*. Does the social network inspire the recipient of the support to feel a sense of mastery in relation to coping with the stressor (Antonucci & Jackson, 1987)? Finally, does the outcome make the person feel more effective? This attribute might be called self-efficacy or perceived self-competence (Bandura, 1977; Weisz & Stipek, 1982).

A problem with research on stress and coping is that linear models are difficult to develop, and components are confounded. How does one distinguish an outcome from a chronic strain? Lupus, for example, could easily qualify as both. Moreover, some psychological syndromes typically thought of as outcomes could become causes of new events (Zautra, 1986); for example, depressed individuals are not a pleasure to be around and may cause a relationship to rupture, thereby starting a new stressful event cycle. Outcomes and appraisals cannot always be distinguished; for example, is caregiver burden best thought about as an appraisal or as an outcome (Zarit, 1989)? Loss of social support can become equivalent to an interpersonal stressor (Zautra, 1986). Psychological attributes may qualify as both outcomes and as mediators; for example, self-esteem and self-efficacy attributions may be both. People are the agents of their own stress through creating chronic strain in their own lives (Maddi, 1989). One form of coping, behavior focused, involves changing the stressor. In brief, despite how it is drawn here, the model must be regarded as transactional or cyclical. The implication for intervention of a cyclical model is that introducing any change can have effects throughout the system described by the model.

The most important point to be made in this chapter is that, without tackling the conceptual and analytical issues, doing responsible intervention is impeded. Planning an intervention requires that the goals, methods, and expected outcomes be defined and understood in relation to some model.

PSYCHOLOGICAL INTERVENTIONS

How can the amalgamated model of stress be combined with a community perspective on psychological intervention? Primary prevention relies on four fundamental strategies: eliminate the stressful event, modify the physical or social environment, strengthen psychological resources and coping skills, and strengthen the social network (Gesten & Jason, 1987). A fifth strategy, inspired by health psychology, is improved health practices, which can keep tension from being as toxic (Maddi, 1989). These five strategies can be mapped onto the amalgamated model of stress and thus begin to provide a taxonomy of interventions (see Figure 11.2).

The following discussion identifies each element of the model and provides some examples. The examples come from research, self-help books such as Nathan, Staats, and Rosch (1987) *The Doctors' Guide to Instant Stress Relief: A Psychological and Medical System,* and clinical experience. The research and clinical examples included here all refer to older adults. Older adults are rarely emphasized in prevention

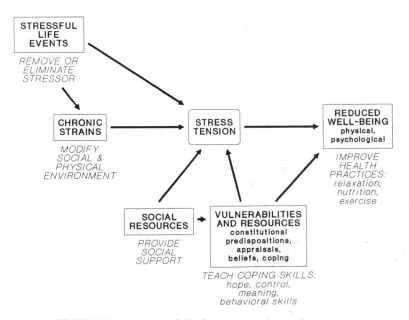

FIGURE 11.2 Model of intervention with stress.

literature, however, and virtually no popular books on stress target the elderly population.

The method of administration imagined in these examples is that there is a professional or paraprofessional helper. The format could be individual, family, or support group. The model could equally well constitute advice to caregivers or could be turned into a self-help book, perhaps called *Stress Management: The Guide to Untarnished Golden Years*. No matter what method or format is used, consistent with the efficacy theme of the model, it is essential for the professional to provide education and choices, not prescriptions.

Removing or Eliminating Stressors

Events over whose occurrence one has control are easiest to prevent, but they may be less stressful than the unexpected event. Even if events cannot be prevented, sometimes they can be scheduled. To the extent that life change is additive, as would be suggested by Holmes and Rahe (1967), then by scheduling events, it is possible to spread out change and reduce stress at any one point in time. For example, it is not necessary for a grandmother to have cataract surgery the same month as her second grandchild is due to arrive. There may be some discretion in scheduling a relocation. Making lists of things to do can reveal opportunities for improved scheduling. In turn, *The Doctors' Guide* suggests that people also compile "Not-To-Do" lists as a way of decreasing number of hassles.

Sometimes stressful events that were not prevented must be quickly eliminated. For example, Sherman (1981) cites the problem of having the heat shut off for nonpayment of a utility bill. In such a case, restoration of heat must be dealt with before any other more psychological type of intervention.

Modifying Social or Physical Environment

Examples of modification of the physical environment include rearranging the furnishings to promote social interaction, making architectural modifications to improve accessibility for those with impairments, and improving the lighting. *The Doctors' Guide* mentions that cluttered surroundings are a reminder of uncompleted tasks, so that removing clutter or finding an uncluttered hideaway can help.

The most typical examples of modifying the social environment involve making isolated people less isolated—for example, setting up telephone networks for the homebound (Evans, Smith, Werkhoven, Fox, & Pritzl, 1986) or organizing a friendly visitors program (Bogat & Jason, 1983). At the same time, it is important not to assume that all isolation is unwanted, and that everyone who spends time alone is lonely (Peplau, Bikson, Rook, & Goodchilds, 1982; Rook, 1984). Placing programs in the context of the model makes their conceptual bases more apparent. A common belief implicitly underlying many activity programs for older adults is that it is good to increase social contacts and interaction. Such an aim requires closer analysis, as it may be inadvertently patronizing if foisted on those for whom activity level was not a chronic strain.

Rodin et al. (1987) have reviewed several environmental interventions in institutions in which inducing greater perceived control resulted in positive outcomes, generally psychological well-being and health. Typically, the environment was restructured to provide residents with more choices or more responsibilities.

Caregiver interventions often include environmental modification, for example, making provision for the caregiver to get out of the house through use of day care, in-home assistance, or respite care. This modification reduces the disruption to other aspects of the caregiver's life, alleviating part of the chronic strain.

Teaching Coping Skills

The bulk of interventions for stress fall under the following coping skills headings: teaching communication skills, training in assertiveness, building a stress-resistant personality, stopping stressful thoughts, engaging in positive thinking, challenging dysfunctional self-evaluations (Nathan et al., 1987; Reinhart & Sargent, 1980; Sherman, 1981). As an example of stopping stressful thinking, a string of thoughts might pop into an older person's mind including "my daughter never visits me," "I can't remember anything anymore," "no one wants to be with someone who can't remember anything," and so on. The individual is instructed to say "stop" to these thoughts while visualizing a large red stop sign. Positive thinking may be encouraged with adages. The older adult might tape a card to the bathroom mirror proclaiming "Live each day as if it was your last because some day you're going to be right" (Nathan et al., 1987).

Rather than seeing any particular categories of coping skills as good and others as bad, the current tendency is to see having a variety of coping skills as most desirable. For example, denial—previously thought to represent ineffectual and immature coping—has been shown to be useful (Horowitz, 1985), probably in combination with some direct problem-solving strategies as well. This approach also permits considering individual differences in preferred styles of coping.

Stress-management classes generally involve teaching people to anticipate events, alter perceptions of events, and enlarge their repertoire of coping skills (Hough, Gongla, Brown, & Goldston, 1985). The idea of anticipating events is deemed particularly relevant to include in interventions for older adults who do have predictable events looming ahead, although at an unknown temporal distance. Sometimes this discussion is facilitated by presenting theories of adult psychosocial development. The purpose of all these stress-management skills is to eliminate self-defeating appraisals, enhance perceived controllability or manageability, and make available a greater variety of ways of handling the nearly inevitable stress.

Reich and Zautra (1989) conducted a controlled evaluation of an intervention designed to increase older adults' sense of control over positive experiences and sense of mastery over negative life events. Sessions were designed to teach recently bereaved or disabled people the difference between events they cause and those they do not, suggest ways of increasing the frequency of self-chosen positive events, and show methods of responding cognitively and behaviorally to externally caused negative events. Reich and Zautra (1989) found some positive effects of the intervention on mental health.

It might well be necessary to consider multiple elements in the model as part of intervening at any particular point. For example, Franzke (1987) concluded that assertion skill training was not an adequate substitute for more community resources for older persons.

Providing Social Support

Several studies have explored types of support and distinguished the more helpful from the less helpful. Lehman, Ellard, and Wortman (1986) found that forced cheerfulness or "I know just how you feel" were not rated helpful by bereaved respondents. Nonetheless, widows did appreciate emotional support, even more than tangible assistance. Others have noted that the idea of "potential help" is very useful; in other words, knowing that there is somewhere to turn if concrete assistance is ever needed.

Support groups are a common vehicle for provision of emotional support and information (i.e., affirmation) and teaching coping skills (Zarit, Orr, & Zarit, 1985) as well as for providing a sense of meaning as group participants become involved in creating community resources and lobbying for changes in policy (Pearlin, Turner, & Semple, 1989). Groups are often specific to a stressful event or situation (e.g., Alzheimer's disease caregivers, stroke patients, or widows).

The literature tends to suggest that supportive intervention following a stressful event or after the onset of a chronic strain is improved by (a) knowing the normal course of resolving the event, (b) anticipating the types of support that might be helpful, and (c) refraining from inadvertent pathologizing of the individual (Gatz & Stacey, in press). For example, to work with spouses of dementia patients requires some knowledge of that disease and the usual reactions of family caregivers. Gerontological research can be informative, and individual differences must be respected. For example, Kasl's chapter in this book suggests that men whose spouse was seriously ill are a uniquely "at-risk" group, and Lieberman's results in this book warn that it would be a mistake to encourage all widows to grieve.

Antonucci and Jackson (1987) have spelled out conceptual implications for intervention by professionals in support networks. Specifically, the goal of the provider of the intervention is to give support in the form of a belief in the ability of the older person to manage the event or stressor. This belief should lead to more optimal coping behavior.

Improving Health Practices

Self-help guides put a lot of emphasis on training your body to relax (Nathan et al., 1987). Proper diet, exercise, and avoiding excessive caffeine and alcohol receive various amounts of play. The "wellness" movement also focuses attention on health practices. Engaging in positive health practices reduces tension and acts directly to improve physical health. As well, because the model is cyclical, relaxing may have an effect on attributions that may mediate chronic stressful circumstances. Relaxation alone is an insufficient stress-management tactic, however. The idea of prevention would argue for starting as far to the left of the model as possible.

CONCLUSION

It should be noticed that concepts of control, self-efficacy, and perceived competence apply across the entire chart and can be used to organize intervention strategies. Successful interventions seem quite consistently to enhance people's feelings of mastery and hope. Efficacy is changed by successful interventions but is also relevant to effecting change (Rodin et al., 1987). Whether the person believes himself or herself capable of managing the stressor is important (i.e., locus-of-control handle). Whether social support and professional interventions are rendered in a fashion that supports or undermines the person's sense of competence is important (support and efficacy process). Whether the person ends up feeling more in charge of his or her own life or demoralized is important. In brief, perceived control is important at every step of the model.

It is argued that any intervention must respect individual differences and thereby the autonomy of the intended recipient. This point is especially salient for older persons who already face many stereotypes and threats to personal autonomy. Apart from any ethical considerations, interventions will not otherwise be effective. This line of thinking leads to a "double-decker" model of control enhancement in which the professional provides information and teaches competencies while letting the intended recipient choose how much responsibility he or she desires or prefers to delegate.

In these ways, through attention to a model of stress and coping, and related considerations of control and autonomy, responsible and effective psychological interventions can be planned that will help older individuals manage the stress that is an inevitable aspect of life.

ACKNOWLEDGMENTS

The author thanks Michele Karel, Miriam Kelly, and Malcolm Klein for constructive comments during the writing of this chapter. Preparation of this chapter was facilitated by grant no. 9 R37 AG07977 from the National Institute on Aging.

REFERENCES

Antonucci, T. C., & Jackson, J. S. (1987). Social support, interpersonal efficacy, and health: A life course perspective. In L. L. Carstensen & B. A. Edelstein (Eds.), *Handbook of clinical gerontology* (pp. 291–311). New York: Pergamon Press.

Bandura, A. (1977). Self-efficacy: Toward a unifying theory of behavioral change. *Psychological Review, 84,* 191–215.

Bloom, B. L. (1985). *Stressful life event theory and research: Implications for primary prevention* (DHHS Publication No. (ADM) 85-1385). Rockville, MD: National Institute of Mental Health.

Bogat, G. A., & Jason, L. A. (1983). An evaluation of two visiting programs for elderly community residents. *International Journal of Aging and Human Development, 17,* 267–280.

Caplan, G. (1964). *Principles of preventive psychiatry.* New York: Basic Books.

Dunkel-Schetter, C., & Wortman, C. B. (1981). Dilemmas of social support: Parallels between victimization and aging. In S. B. Kiesler, J. N. Morgan, & V. K. Oppenheimer (Eds.), *Aging: Social change* (pp. 349–381). New York: Academic Press.

Evans, R. L., Smith, K. M., Werkhoven, W. S., Fox, H. R., & Pritzl, D. O. (1986). Cognitive telephone group therapy with physically disabled elderly persons. *The Gerontologist, 26,* 8–11.

Felton, B. J. (1982). The aged: Settings, services, and needs. In L. R. Snowden (Ed.), *Reaching the underserved: Mental health needs of neglected populations* (pp. 23–42). Beverly Hills, CA: Sage.

Franzke, A. W. (1987). The effects of assertiveness training on older adults. *The Gerontologist, 27,* 13–16.

Gatz, M., Popkin, S. J., Pino, C. D., & VandenBos, G. R. (1985). Psychological interventions with older adults. In J. E. Birren & K. W. Schaie (Eds.), *Handbook of the psychology of aging* (2nd ed., pp. 755–785). New York: Van Nostrand Reinhold.

Gatz, M., Siegler, I. C., George, L. K., & Tyler, F. B. (1986). Attributional components of locus of control: Longitudinal, retrospective, and contemporaneous analyses. In M. M. Baltes & P. B. Baltes (Eds.), *The psychology of control and aging* (pp. 237–263). Hillsdale, NJ: Erlbaum.

Gatz, M., & Stacey, C. (in press). Community and preventive interventions for normative occurrences of later life. In J. Rappaport & E. Seidman (Eds.), *Handbook of community psychology.* New York: Plenum.

Gesten, E. L., & Jason, L. A. (1987). Social and community interventions. *Annual review of psychology, 38,* 427–460.

Holmes, T. H., & Rahe, R. H. (1967). The Social Readjustment Rating Scale. *Journal of Psychosomatic Research, 11,* 213–218.

Horowitz, M. J. (1985). Psychological responses to stress: The stress response syndromes. In H. H. Goldman & S. E. Goldston (Eds.), *Preventing stress-related psychiatric disorders* (DHHS Publication No. (ADM) 85-1366, pp. 107–147). Rockville, MD: National Institute of Mental Health.

Hough, R. L., Gongla, P. A., Brown, V. B., & Goldston, S. E. (1985). *Psychiatric epidemiology and prevention: The possibilities.* Papers resulting from a research planning workshop held through the Neuropsychiatric Institute, Los Angeles. University of California, Los Angeles.

Hultsch, D. F., & Plemons, J. K. (1979). Life events and life-span development. In P. B. Baltes & O. G. Brim, Jr. (Eds.), *Life-span development and behavior* (Vol. 2, pp. 1–36). New York: Academic Press.

Kahn, R. L., & Antonucci, T. C. (1981). Convoys of social support: A life course approach. In S. B. Kiesler, J. N. Morgan, & V. K. Oppenheimer (Eds.), *Aging: Social change* (pp. 383–405). New York: Academic Press.

Lasoski, M. C. (1986). Reasons for low utilization of mental health services by the elderly. In T. L. Brink (Ed.), *Clinical gerontology: A guide to assessment and intervention* (pp. 1–18). New York: Haworth Press.

Lazarus, R. S., & Folkman, S. (1984). Coping and adaptation. In W. D. Gentry (Ed.), *Handbook of behavioral medicine* (pp. 282–325). New York: Guilford.

Lehman, D. R., Ellard, J. H., & Wortman, D. B. (1986). Social support for the bereaved: Recipients' and providers' perspectives on what is helpful. *Journal of Consulting and Clinical Psychology, 54,* 438–446.

Lieberman, M. A. (1975). Adaptive processes in late life. In N. Datan & L. H. Ginsberg (Eds.), *Life-span developmental psychology: Normative life crises* (pp. 135–159). New York: Academic Press.

Maddi, S. (1989, April). *Issues in stress mastery: The hardiness approach.* Colloquium presented at University of Southern California, Los Angeles.

Moos, R. H., & Billings, A. G. (1982). Conceptualizing and measuring coping resources and processes. In L. Goldberger & S. Breznitz (Eds.), *Handbook of stress: Theoretical and clinical aspects* (pp. 212–230). New York: Free Press.

Murrell, S. A., Norris, F. H., & Grote, C. (1987). Life events in older adults. In L. H. Cohen (Ed.), *Life events and psychological functioning: Theoretical and methodological issues* (pp. 96–122). Beverly Hills: Sage.

Nathan, R. G., Staats, T. E., & Rosch, P. J. (1987). *The doctor's guide to instant stress relief: A psychological and medical system.* New York: Putnam.

Norris, F. H., & Murrell, S. A. (1988). Prior experience as a moderator of disaster impact on anxiety symptoms in older adults. *American Journal of Community Psychology, 16,* 665–683.

Pearlin, L. I. (1989). The sociological study of stress. *Journal of Health and Social Behavior, 30,* 241–256.

Pearlin, L. I., Turner, H., & Semple, S. (1989). Coping and the mediation of caregiver stress. In E. Light & B. D. Lebowitz (Eds.), *Alzheimer's disease treatment and family stress: Directions for research* (DHHS Publication No. (ADM) 89-1569, pp. 198–217). Rockville, MD: National Institute of Mental Health.

Peplau, L. A., Bikson, T. K., Rook, K. S., & Goodchilds, J. D. (1982). Being old and living alone. In L. A. Peplau & D. Perlman (Eds.), *Loneliness: A sourcebook of current theory, research and therapy* (pp. 327–347). New York: Wiley Interscience.

Reich, J. W., & Zautra, A. J. (1989). A perceived control intervention for at-risk older adults. *Psychology and Aging, 4,* 415–424.

Reinhart, R. A., & Sargent, S. S. (1980). The humanistic approach: The Ventura County creative aging workshops. In S. S. Sargent (Ed.), *Non-traditional therapy and counseling with the aging* (pp. 163–177). New York: Springer.

Rodin, J., Cashman, C., & Desiderato, L. (1987). Intervention and aging: Enrichment and prevention. In M. W. Riley, J. D. Matarazzo, & A. Baum (Eds.), *Perspectives in behavioral medicine: The aging dimension* (pp. 149–172). Hillsdale, NJ: Erlbaum.

Rook, K. S. (1984). Interventions for loneliness: A review and analysis. In L. A. Peplau & S. E. Goldston (Eds.), *Preventing the harmful consequences of severe and persistent loneliness* (DHHS Publication No. (ADM) 85-1312, pp. 47–79). Rockville, MD: National Institute of Mental Health.

Sherman, E. A. (1981). *Counseling the aging: An integrative approach.* New York: Free Press.

Thoits, P. A. (1986). Social support as coping assistance. *Journal of Consulting and Clinical Psychology, 54,* 416–423.

Weisz, J. R., & Stipek, D. J. (1982). Competence, contingency, and the development of perceived control. *Human Development, 25,* 250–281.

Zarit, S. H. (1989). Issues and directions in family intervention research. In E. Light & B. D. Lebowitz (Eds.), *Alzheimer's disease treatment and family stress: Directions for research* (DHHS Publication No. (ADM) 89-1569, pp. 458–486). Rockville, MD: National Institute of Mental Health.

Zarit, S. H., Orr, N. K., & Zarit, J. M. (1985). *The hidden victims of Alzheimer's disease: Families under stress.* New York: New York University Press.

Zautra, A. J. (1986). *Third generation life event research on high risk older adults.* Colloquium presented at University of Southern California, Los Angeles.

12

Family-Based Long-Term Care for the Elderly: Stress Considerations

Thomas H. Walz and Pamela Brown

There is little debate about the policy significance of long-term care of the elderly today. It is indeed one of the major social and economic issues facing the nation. Three key factors help to explain the rise of long-term care's policy significance: (a) the changing demographics of society, (b) the technological changes occurring in health delivery, and (c) the expanding role of the professions and the marketplace in the delivery of long-term care. Each of these factors has contributed to a scale of long-term care that is becoming more costly than the nation may be able or willing to afford.

The elderly population in the United States is now larger and older than at any previous time in history. At the turn of the century there were only 3 million people 65 years or older, approximately 4% of the total U.S. population. Aging was thought to be a biological process, and the care of the elderly, other than complex medical services, was provided within the family. For those without families and in poverty surrogate care was available only in poor farms or old folks' homes.

By the year 2000, a little more than a decade away, it is estimated that the number of persons 65 years and older will be 35 million, or slightly more than 13% of the population (Zopf, 1986). This increment in the absolute number of the elderly will continue until 2015 when the numbers jump sharply as the "baby boomers" of the 1950s to 1960s begin to reach their seniority. Hosts of long-term care providers who did not exist a decade ago now dot the landscape. More providers can be expected as the number of elderly and the complexity of long-term care increases.

The long-term care impact of this demographic shift comes because of the increase in life expectancy and the expanded period of protracted dependency the elderly experience. Life expectancy has increased 6 years since midcentury. The years of dependent care may extend into decades for some elders.

Both formal and informal responses to long-term care similarly are undergoing change. Who responds and how they respond follows a complex network of policy choices. Today's policy framework for dealing with the long-term care of the elderly is affected by the current technological imperative in health care and the expanded role of government and the marketplace in dealing with the health needs of the elderly. Public policy simply follows the lines of an advanced capitalist political economy, with its heavy high technology bias and its growing welfare-state component.

The consequences of pursuing such a policy direction is becoming increasingly evident. The formal provider system role in long-term care grows and with it a continuing shift toward heavier technology-dependent care. The informal provider system remains, but with some role loss or displacement and with limited economic support for its continuing contributions. The outcome of this development has been a rapid rise in the cost of long-term care for the elderly. By 1990, an estimated $55 billion annually will be expended for nursing home care alone of the elderly (General Accounting Office, 1986).

It would appear that the fiscal crisis associated with paying for long-term care of the elderly will lead to consideration of alternative approaches to long-term care. The family-based approach presented here is one such alternative. As an alternative it does have major consequences for stress in the family.

In this chapter we explore the family-based approach as a potential policy development. After defining the approach, we discuss some of the issues surrounding its feasibility and implementation. Of central concern is the readiness or preparedness of the family to take on even greater responsibility for the long-term care of its members. As a special focus of this chapter we then explore in some depth the "stress impact" on the family that a family-based approach could produce. We end by exploring funding and implementation issues that the family-based approach could present.

DEFINITION OF FAMILY-BASED APPROACH

A family-based approach to long-term care views the family as the primary institution for the care and nurture of its members. The family is seen as the normative and accepted unit for general caregiving of the elderly. As the central caregiving institution for the elderly, the family ideally should be able to expand and adapt to fit the changing dependency needs of the aged person. Even complex caregiving tasks should not be rejected as being necessarily outside the competency of the family.

In a family-based approach to long-term care, the formal health and social service agencies have a place. Their roles, however, are considered secondary or supplementary to the family. Formal providers are not viewed as replacements to family caregiving except in exceptional circumstances. When care has been given over to one or more of these formal providers, it is expected that they involve the family as much as possible in caregiving.

Family-based care should be clearly differentiated from community-based care. Community-based care typically is provider oriented and often results in "taking over" caregiving from a family. Service imperialism is seen as a real threat to family-based development. This is especially true in profit agencies. The private long-term care market seeks "business" (Select Committee on Aging, 1986). The less care the family provides for itself, the more it must seek from the market. The informal and formal sectors can find themselves in direct competition in providing long-term care to the elderly.

The family-based approach builds on the reality that fully three fourths of all long-term care is currently provided by the family (Brody, 1985). The approach assumes the family to be basically interested in providing care and in protecting its nurturing and caregiving role in society. It further assumes that the family is capable of handling the task.

The family is seen as a social and economic unit capable of expanding or contracting its functions depending on how societal resources and rewards are distributed. Families are also assumed to be in a constant state of development—capable of learning. Even in instances in which long-term caregivng demands are complex, the family is viewed as capable of learning to handle the more complicated needs of their older members.

Definition of Family

In defining family-based care, we must also share our definition of family. Family, in our view, is an identifiable network of persons, often but not necessarily blood related, whose bond includes a commitment to sharing of resources, exchange of affective relations, and the provision of mutual support. The unit can be as small as a couple and as large as a kibbutz. Dychtwald & Flower (1989) perhaps best captures this changing definition of family in their new book Age Wave: The Challenges and Opportunities of an Aging America.

Evaluation of Family Capability

As with all societal institutions, the family has experienced great changes in the 20th century. The nuclear family of the industrial epoch has given way to the micronuclear family and its variants of the new postindustrial period. The new family is smaller, less capable, more mobile, more divided geographically, less interdependent economically and less bound by traditional blood ties (Levitan & Belous, 1981).

The family of today is also characterized by greater variation than ever before. Naisbitt (1982) cites 13 accepted forms of family in America today. Consequently, generalizations about the family with respect to long-term caregiving will be difficult.

It has been charged that filial piety is severely eroded in today's family. Self-interest is believed to drive our "now" families. Just as families often avoid child-rearing responsibilities, so many will avoid caring for their frail aged members. Research, however, does not support this commonly held belief (Brody, 1981; Shanas, 1979). Numerous studies suggest that the family abandonment thesis is grossly overstated. There remains considerable contact between the elderly and their families.

Even if there is family willingness to do the long-term care job, however, is the family equipped to do so? After all, the elderly now require more extended, complex long-term care assistance at a time when the family itself seems stripped of many essential resources. The family membership rarely includes trained specialists in the health and social care fields.

Families today are clearly smaller than in the past because of greatly reduced birthrates (Levitan & Belous, 1981). In Europe, America, and Japan birthrates have fallen well below the 2.1 child to family ratio needed for population replacement. In the long run this can have serious effects on sustaining both the social security and long-term care systems (Adams, 1988). The retired ideally depend on a sizable strong work force for their support. Conversely, fewer children also means that time and money expenses for dependent children could be reallocated to the long-term care of the elderly. Likewise, a more adult population assures more adult resources for caregiving—at least up to the period of the aging of the boom population group.

There is little question about the current instability of the conventional family. At current rates half of all American marriages begun in the early 1980s will end up in divorce (Cherlin & Furstenberg, Jr., 1983). Although remarriage typically follows the breakup of marriage, extended periods of single parenthood are common (Levitan & Belous, 1981). Remarriage, when it occurs, creates the phenomenon of the blended family. In both instances, the long-term caregiving capacity of the family may be strained. In multiple marriages, traditional ties to parents or in-laws may become less clear. Filial responsibility must be redefined, or at least reconfirmed.

What we may be witnessing in the instability of the conventional family system is not necessarily a full-scale destabilization of all of the new emerging family systems. As the older persons recognize that they may not be able to depend as much on their children, their loyalties and ties may shift to neighbors, friends, and a new network of significant others (Dychtwald & Flower, 1989). Mutual aid may still go on but between a different set of individuals. There are also many more remarriages today among the elderly themselves, especially those who have been widowed.

In an aging family system in many rural areas, elderly persons may have to turn to brothers and sisters rather than children and grandchildren for their long-term care assistance. Youth unfortunately is fast abandoning the rural areas in America. Friends and neighbors, at least in stable communities, likewise appear to assume similar roles in both urban and rural areas.

The mobility pattern of family members has influenced family caregiving capabilities. Visiting an ailing aged parent from a thousand miles away is costly in both time and money. Although we often think of the young family member moving out and away from the aging members, the reverse is also true. The retirement patterns of many elderly may lead them away from their children, former friends, and neighbors.

Patterns of mobility also allow for a return to a family homestead as well as away from it. Some members do return when caregiving needs require it. How common this pattern may be is not well documented.

The instability of the family often overshadows the stability of the marriages of today's elderly cohort. Never have so many golden weddings been celebrated in human history. Caregiving provided spouse to spouse is the bedrock of today's informal long-term care system. This caregiving arrangement has been extended through the added years to life. Children rarely take over as caregivers until one of the spouses dies or grows too infirm to care for the other. This pattern may change in the future as the subsequent cohorts of elderly come out of the marriage-divorce-remarriage go-round.

Likewise, living longer still favors women. Women not only end up having to take on the spouse caregiver role, but her added years may leave her without her own spouse caregiver in her frailty period. There are many sides to the family destabilization scenario.

The family living environment is in the midst of transformation. The single-family home is fast becoming an arrangement of the past. Apartments and condos, even in rural areas, are taking over as the prototype family homestead. The most commonly sold housing unit in America is the mobile home. Changes in family habitat create some additional barriers to elderly family caregiving. Families cannot bring a parent or relative to live with them unless place and space permit. The changing family habitat is an additional reason why so many elderly live "alone."

Perhaps the main change in family structure that affects the long-term care of the elderly has been the rise of "dual careerism" in the family. With both husband and wife working full- or part-time, there are few time and energy resources left at home for caregiving. It has been the older adult woman in the family who has been the principal caregiver (Brody, 1979). It is also the older woman who has shown the greatest increase in labor-force participation. Fully four out of five adult women in America are in the work force today. Many, of course, also double as caregivers to a frail relative (Brody, Johnsen,

Fulcomer, & Lang, 1983). Others have had to yield this responsibility to surrogate caregivers.

The profile of the older woman at work, sometimes doubling as caregiver, raises some interesting questions. As with younger women with children in the workplace, care arrangements for a dependent have to be worked out. The work of women often yields modest returns, whereas child or adult care can be costly. The net addition to the family income from outside work is often minimal, albeit essential.

Ironically, the older woman worker may end up in a "service job" at minimum wages—such as nurse's aide work in a nursing home. This is approximately the same type work she would do if she remained at the home. There are, of course, many reasons for working outside the home. The need for different type of "work" may not be one of them. Money is not always the reason either.

This scenario suggests that the caregivers are out there. The question is where do we want them and where would they prefer to be—at home or in the workplace? Likewise there is no defensible reason why the family caregiver must be a woman. The potential family caregiving pool has a large male component. Many older men have been displaced from or bear a tenuous relationship to stable employment, especially in the last decade of their work life. Many would be theoretically available to assume a family caregiver role.

The analysis of the changing family indicates that despite some structural alterations and functional shifts in the family, the family remains a resource with yet untapped potential in the long-term care of the elderly.

Family Integrity Argument

In the days of bottom-line economic approaches to public policy issues, an argument about long-term caregiving rarely heard is the family integrity argument. We have witnessed in recent years an incredible encroachment of family functions by other social institutions. Health, education, and welfare organizations have all laid title to a variety of service needs that the family has historically provided to itself—child care, early child socialization, primary health care, general counseling, recreation and the like. Long-term care is threatening to become yet another province of the nonfamily institutions.

It is difficult to imagine a strong, viable family system that does not maintain control over critical and vital functions (e.g., economic, health, and welfare) of its members. If the family is just a collection of individuals whose needs are met outside the family unit, why have a family unit at all? Some believe that the increase of divorce, separation, and single parenthood is associated with the lack of essentiality of a stable family system.

A belief in a strong viable family system could require one to rethink the role of the family in long-term care. No matter the burden, if families are to retain control over later life dependency, dying, and death they must fight to remain central in long-term caregiving. The family-based approach provides the philosophy and methodology for maintaining family integrity in this area. The family life cycle and the critical events within each cycle, in our opinion, should remain under family auspices and control. In a postindustrial age in which the economic function of the family is less vital to societal survival, the noneconomic roles of families need to take on even greater prominence. Long-term caregiving is one of these important functions.

It is evident that it is in the state's interest to encourage and support a strong family system. As a collective of healthy families, the state can be only strengthened. To build up the "welfare state" at the expense of the family makes no sense at all. In the long run, it is probably not even affordable. The market system is a real competitor to the family. Government support of the market system has been substantial. For the family to remain competitive, it needs balanced public support.

Stress Considerations

The central issue in this chapter is the stress considerations to the family that a family-based approach to long-term care could present. The literature is replete with data showing that family caregiving can be stressful (Brody, 1985). The discussion on changes occurring within the family system also suggests that families have become even more vulnerable to caregiver stress. Working outside the home, declining personal incomes, and unstable marriages could make caring for aging adults an unwelcome, highly burdensome task.

As proponents of family-based care, we will examine the defense that can be made to the assertion that taking on greater long-term care responsibilities necessarily results in more stress or bad stress. By bad stress, we mean the kind of stress that eats away at the personal health of the caregiver.

The literature makes it clear that not all stress is bad (Brody, 1985). Caring for an aged dependent may be vitally important to a caregiver's sense of self-worth and well-being. In a study of family caregivers of the elderly in Iowa, the authors found that when asked if they would do it all over again (provide long-term care for an adult relative), the family caregivers almost universally said they would. The key to wearing stress well seemed to be recognition and regard by others for doing the job (Walz & Reese, 1983).

The current pattern of working outside the home (in lieu of caregiving) does not necessarily eliminate stress in a "former" caregiver. The person at work may experience stress associated with guilt at not doing the caregiving job or doing it poorly as a result of trying to combine the responsibility of a job with caregiving tasks. For some being away at work means being in a state of worry about a loved one left at home alone or left in the care of another in which one may not have full confidence. In addition, being at work means also being at risk for work-related stress. One can end up trading one set of stresses for another.

Long-term caregiving also could be looked on as having stress-reducing potential. Estranged children and parents, even spouses, can be reunited through the caregiving relationship. The positive feelings of service to another can be a stress reducer, especially for those individuals who have been natural caregivers all their lives. The sense of purpose that comes from having another's life in your hands may be particularly important to people whose opportunities in other areas may have been limited.

Increases in stress as a result of family caregivers come from a variety of new sources. Home care is both becoming more complex and of longer duration. Taking on a difficult task is usually manageable if it does not last a long time. Until recently death occurred relatively soon after a loss of independency. This is less true today. Stress that is manageable on a day-to-day basis can become overwhelming over the long haul.

The complexity of care issue has been already felt as a result of the diagnostic-related–group cost-containment strategy in Medicare. Getting aged persons back home sicker and quicker simply shifts more care to the family. The care demands are usually more complex because the patient is sicker and their medical needs greater. In the family-based approach it is suggested that family members can be trained to take on more sophisticated and responsible medical or home health management procedures. This could occasion added stress for the caregiver.

Such stress could be offset by a somewhat closer articulation of the family caregiver with selected formal agency supports. When it is recognized that the family is attempting to take on the bulk of caregiving, professionals need to present themselves more as supporters of caregivers, not their replacement.

Economic stress is felt in many families today. This is often the reason why traditional family caregivers are being driven into the workplace when they may not wish to do so. The high costs of formal long-term may make it necessary to continue providing care even while working outside the home. Some prevention of stress resulting from economic insufficiency or insecurity could come from greater public economic support to caregiving families. In the conclusion of this chapter we explore some of these economic considerations.

Any difficult task, especially a task that is protracted, can lead to cumulative stress. In these situations stress can only be reduced through respite from that task. A family-based approach to long-term care without a good system of respite care could prove disastrous. Adult day care, day hospitals, vacation-time respites, and short daily respites all need to be planned for if family-based care is not to overwhelm family caregivers. As yet no system of respite care for elderly dependents has developed in the United States.

A factor to consider in stress management is the variation in stress thresholds among individuals. One reason why some long-term caregivers manage well is their foreknowledge of what is involved in dependent adult caregiving and knowledge of the way illnesses manifest themselves. Fear of the unknown is a major precipitator of stress. So any preparation, education, and anticipatory guidance provided a family caregiver could have substantial stress-reducing qualities. In the plan for operationalizing a family-based approach, we discuss strategies for assuring that such preventative education is provided to the family caregiver.

Overall, the family-based approach does present conditions for stress to occur in the caregivers. The approach, however, is designed to build in supports and incentives to reduce, limit, or offset any added stress occasioned by taking on more of the long-term caregiving role.

Economics Considerations

The argument has been repeatedly made that alternatives to expensive institutional care of the elderly should be cost saving. The promotion of community-based care was touted as a cost-saving measure. Health Care Finance Administration (HCFA) has been skeptical, however, and has held back wholesale funding of community-based care. As it appears to be turning out, community-based care can be very expensive, particularly if federal funds are available through medical waivers (General Accounting Office, 1982). Would this not also be the case with family-based alternatives?

Within the family-based model, economic incentives to families willing to assume major long-term care demands are envisioned. Because informal care has traditionally been free, this would be a new long-term care cost. Another incentive to families is to provide them more help and support from formal agencies in doing the long-term care job. A strengthened family system, however, probably would make even greater demands on selected parts of the community care system (e.g., adult day care, respite care, etc.). Family members as advocates for long-term care could be expected to make greater use of health and social services on behalf of their elderly relative. This would be particularly true if, under the family-based approach, caregivers were given training as advocates and case managers.

Conversely, if families did more of what agencies do, then the dollars needed for the formal long-term care provider system should be less. Even if the total volume of service demand remained static, costs should drop because families are less expensive, with less overhead than agencies. Overall, it would appear that the informal system could do its part of the long-term care job far cheaper than most formal agencies. The issue remains how to reverse trends. How much of what the formal agencies now do could or would the family, if properly rewarded and trained, be willing and able to "take back"?

The actual costs of the family-based approach depend on many variables. Not the least of these is how much direct financial "incentive" could be provided to the family caregivers (Arling & McAuley, 1983).

An economic incentive that does not require a transfer of funds is the awareness that by providing long-term care to a family member, the family is earning some protection of the relative's estate. Too often these days estates are rapidly spent once the elder gets caught up in high-cost health and nursing home care.

Financing the family-based approach would necessitate some major adjustments in Medicare and Medicaid funding. To date neither federal program has been generously willing to fund other than basic doctor-driven medical care. Reluctantly, however, both programs have expanded support for some community-based services (e.g., hospice, day care, etc.). Medicaid waivers have been the usual means of paying for these expansions (Doty, Lieu, & Wiener, 1985). It is also through the Medicaid waiver arrangements that payment to families in some states for some caregiving function has occurred. Such waivers, unfortunately, are few and far between. For the family-based approach to develop, additional consideration needs to be given to providing economic incentives to families willing to take on the assignment.

In addition to Medicaid waivers that would allow Medicaid funds to be spent on family care, changes are needed in the Supplemental Security Income (SSI) program, which currently reduces (SSI) benefits for beneficiaries living with family or relatives. Also helpful would be an improved tax deduction for dependent care of an elderly person—one that more truly reflects the actual costs of care.

The Older American Act and Title XX dollars both could be directed toward support of aspects of "family-based care." Chore service and homemaker service funding clearly could include payments to family members. States could use their own appropriations to pilot and underwrite family-based demonstration projects. The state of Iowa for many years has had an elderly care program in which state appropriations are used to supplement purchase of home health care, homemaker service, and adult day care. Unfortunately, only provider agencies have been eligible for these funds.

Although the United States has never adopted a "dependent elders' allowance" concept, the program in countries like France and Canada appears to have been successful. Based on the child allowance model, it is a concept worthy of exploration. Under such a program, any family providing "substantial" or full care of an elderly member would receive a monthly allowance to cover partially expenses associated with that care. Subsidies to rich families would be recovered through the progressive income tax structures, as allowances would need to be declared as income.

The reluctance to fund families for long-term care comes from two concerns: the reluctance to pay families for what they should be expected to do anyway, and the difficulty of monitoring the "service."

How often might we end up paying families for doing nothing? Close monitoring, conversely, tends to push the administrative costs up to the point that it would be actually cheaper to fund "agencies" to do surrogate family work. The state of Illinois chose to suspend its payments to family caregivers for this reason.

A family-based approach need not necessarily be seen as an economic alternative with comparative costs and benefits. A family approach could be implemented as a philosophy using many non-monetary incentives. It could be used to provide competition to the voracious market appetites of the formal agency long-term care providers if nothing else. Society needs to be periodically reminded who in fact is providing the bulk of long-term caregiving at present. It seems ironic that to get someone to clean the apartment of a frail old person it should cost $10 per hour—$5 paid to the homemaker and $5 for administrative overload. Would not it make economic sense to give a few dollars to the family for doing the same task?

Clearly the economics of a family-based model are yet to be tested. Our argument is only that the time has come to put it to the test.

Operationalization of Family-Based Approach

Perhaps the "aging network" would be the best place to locate the administration of a family-based long-term care system. A local agency could be established to help families identify and assess their long-term care needs and plan for a family approach to meeting them. The local unit could help families identify knowledge and skill gaps, and arrange for appropriate training and supervision to carry out selected long-term care tasks that may in the past have been done by professionals or paraprofessionals.

Many of the community-based long-term care agencies would be asked to trade their direct service function for an indirect teaching role. They would have a reduced service profile in many families. The Administration on Aging (AOA) would need to advocate on behalf of families and their capabilities to do the long-term care job. The local agency could serve as a conduit for some financing of family-provided services (using chore or homemaker dollars, albeit through Older Americans Act, Title XX, or Medicaid appropriations).

The local family-based unit could also develop family support groups and, on occasion, help to develop family cooperative approaches to respite, adult day care and home visitations, telephone reassurance, and even nursing home care.

The institutional-based long-term care services, particularly the nursing home, could be encouraged to work more "cooperatively" with families, perhaps offering economic inducements for volunteer aid. The so-called service credits earned through volunteer service and that can be applied to costs of care are examples of what needs to be more fully developed. Nursing homes with high volunteer ratios, perhaps, could be allowed to have lower staff-patient ratios, hence lowering the cost of nursing care.

Family replacements of nonprofessional care (e.g., basic homemaker and chore services) seems entirely feasible—assuming the availability of a family resource. It is only when a more complex medical service is needed that real debate may occur about the family's capacity to provide such a service. Insulin injections, medication administration, bathing of bed sores, tending to open wounds, and physical rehabilitation exercises are types of interventions for which we have felt professional competency is needed. Yet in our operational planning, we would envision that, when motivated, family members should be permitted to be trained in providing such long-term care services. Both teaching and supervision could eventually come from those technically trained. The local family-based service unit would attempt to both encourage and coordinate such efforts.

There is clearly precedent for a family-based approach to the long-term care of the elderly. The approach has been successfully implemented in the child care field, where a wholesale change in child welfare approaches is under way (Bryce, 1979). No longer are children routinely "saved" from their families. Even troubled families are approached as principal resources and institutions for child care. The welfare agency is now a resource for families, not a replacement for families. Family-based long-term care seems to be a concept whose time has come. As a concept there is much to be worked out in its operationalization. This will not come, however, until the concept and philosophy have gained both popular support and public–policy-maker backing. Family-based long-term care is at this stage of development.

Long-term care is truly at a crossroads. One direction is the continued professionalization of care and the medicalization of dying. The other is family-based long-term care, in which the family returns as the primary care unit for the elderly and views dying and death as a stage of human development rather than a medical event.

Family long-term caregiving can be complex, burdensome, and stress inducing. Stress management and prevention in family caregiving of the elderly must remain a major component of a systematic approach to long-term care.

REFERENCES

Adams, P. (1988, February). *Children as contributions in-kind: Integrating social security with family policy.* Paper presented at the annual program meeting of the Council of Social Work, Chicago, IL.

Arling, G., & McAuley, W. (1983). The feasibility of public payments for family caregiving. *The Gerontologist, 23,* 300–306.

Brody, E. (1979, October 27). Women's changing roles, the aging family and long term care of older people. *National Journal,* 1832.

Brody, E. (1981). "Women in the middle" and family help to older people. *Gerontologist, 21,* 471–480.

Brody, E. (1985). Parent care as normative family stress. *The Gerontologist, 25,* 19–29.

Brody, E., Johnsen, P. T., Fulcomer, M. C., & Lang, A. M. (1983). Women's changing roles and help to elderly parents: Attitudes of three generations of women. *Journal of Gerontology, 38,* 597–607.

Bryce, M. (1979). Home-based care: Development and rationale. In S. Maybanks, & M. Bryce (Eds.), *Home-based services for children and families: Policy, practice, & research* (pp. 13–26). Springfield, IL: Charles C Thomas.

Cherlin, A., & Furstenberg, F., Jr. (1983, June). The American family. *Futurist, 2,* 7.

Doty, P., Lieu, K., & Wiener, J. (1985). An overview of long-term care. *Health Care Financing Review, 7,* 42.

Dychtwald, K., & Flower, J. (1989). *Age wave: The challenges and opportunities of an aging America.* Los Angeles: Tarcher.

General Accounting Office. (1982). *The elderly should benefit from expanded home health care, but increasing service will not insure cost reduction* (Publication No. GAO/IPE 83-1). Washington, DC: U.S. Government Printing Office.

General Accounting Office. (1986). *Meeting the needs of the elderly while responding to rising federal costs* (Publication No. GAO/HRD 86-135). Washington, DC: U.S. Government Printing Office.

Levitan, S., & Belous, R. (1981). *What's happening to the American family?* Baltimore, MD: Johns Hopkins Press.

Naisbitt, J. (1982). *Megatrends: Ten new directions transforming our lives.* New York: Warner Communcations.

Select Committee on Aging. (1986). *The black box of home care quality* (Committee Publication No. 99-573). Washington, DC: Congress House Select Committee on Aging.

Shanas, E. (1979). Social myth as hypothesis: The case of the family relations of old people. *The Gerontologist, 19*, 3-9.

Walz, T., & Reese, D. (1983). Intergenerational caregivers of the frail elderly. *Journal of Gerontological Social Work, 5*, 21-34.

Zopf, P. E., Jr. (1986). *America's older population.* Houston, TX: Cap and Gown Press.

Epilogue
Stress Research and Aging: Complexities, Ambiguities, Paradoxes, and Promise

Eva Kahana

The success of scientific discussion lies as much in framing questions that can generate new research as in providing answers to questions previously raised. To highlight some of the fundamental issues explored in this book on stress, health, and aging, this overview is organized around some basic questions put as Alice may have asked them in Wonderland if she were interested in exploring the world of stress research. The answers suggested are both real, controversial, and tongue-in-cheek. Some of the questions posed have been noted or addressed in individual chapters within this book, whereas others point the way to as yet unexplored areas of stress research as applied to the elderly.

WHERE DO STRESSFUL LIFE EVENTS COME FROM AND DO THEY JUST RANDOMLY HAPPEN TO PEOPLE?

Little attention has been directed in stress literature toward understanding systematic influences that affect the amount and type of stress experienced by the elderly. In traditional stress research, focusing on both younger and older populations, stress is typically conceptualized and measured in the form of recent life events. Such events generally comprise the independent variables in studies of stress, based on assumptions that these are random and noncontingent events that reflect environmental presses or stimuli. We are prone to think of the elderly as "finding themselves" in situations that create stress through losses or excessive demands placed on them such as forced retirement or the need to become a caregiver to a frail spouse. Yet even this very expectation bespeaks a hypothesis about the effects of age on stress. Accordingly, it is useful to understand how personal background of the elderly may systematically impact on the likelihood of experiencing specific life events or other stressors.

In addition to demographic factors such as age, sex, and race, which are likely to influence the experience of stressful life events, there also appears to be a relationship between earlier stresses predisposing older adults to experiencing later stress and between one form of stress predisposing individuals to experience another. In addition, prior and current resources including coping and social supports also impact the types of stresses reported by the elderly. Baldwin's focus in this book on contextual and environmental influences on stress experiences of older adults represents a particularly useful direction for understanding factors that impact on late-life stress.

Consideration of stressful life events as discrete singular occurrences represents a further conceptual weakness in the field. In fact, most major stressful life situations present repetitive or even ongoing stresses. Diverse definitions of stress do not describe unrelated phenomena. Gatz's chapter in this book on interventions aptly points out that life events such as death of a spouse are directly related to the chronic strains attendant to being a widow. Thus, it poses a challenge to stress researchers to develop conceptual and operational models that permit an understanding of the interconnectedness among different aspects and sources of stress, and permit exploring antecedents as well as outcomes of diverse stress.

Research on elderly Holocaust survivors reported by Boaz Kahana confirms that systematic influences shape life events of the elderly. Older Holocaust survivors who endured extreme trauma earlier in life report more recent health-related negative life events, while at the same time reporting fewer family-oriented events when compared with a nontraumatized group. Furthermore, he suggests that reduced incidence of problems with children may in fact reflect the high level of family cohesiveness that this group obtains. The latter may be a successful effort at coping with loss of kin experienced by survivors during a critical period of their life-span development.

Close scrutiny of our independent variable in stress research is thus indicated. Consideration of systematic influences on stress opens up new vistas in gerontological research. Thus, we might take seriously the question: Where do life events come from? We may recognize that the answer is not "from thin air."

IS STRESS IN THE EYES OF THE BEHOLDER?

The focus on appraisal and attribution has been an increasingly useful area in stress research (Folkman & Lazarus, 1980). It has helped demonstrate that there are great individual differences in what is or is not defined as stressful. The rich literature on the role of appraisals has called attention to the importance of the interpretive context of stress. Appraisals are seen as critical for determining whether an experience or stimulus is viewed as stressful by the individual. Stress researchers now recognize that it may be foolhardy to have a group of judges determine the readjustment required by a specific life event in a way that would meaningfully apply to a given older individual.

Paralleling emphasis on perceived stress as a critical influence on outcomes, perceived support has also been recognized as a useful approach to conceptualizing buffers in the stress paradigm. Specifically, it has been argued that satisfaction with support may be more important for diminishing adverse sequelae of stress than connectedness to a support network or even objective support received (Wethington & Kessler, 1986). Several of the presentations at this conference underscored the importance of appraisals. I consider it refreshing to note that some counterpoints to the appraisal-based view of stress have also been raised.

The general assumption made in the stress field is that life changes represent negative or potentially harmful stimuli. Pearlin has aptly pointed to the need for specifying exactly what it is that we find stressful about change. He used the example of loss to suggest the need for specifying exactly what is threatened or impacted by a loss. Is it honor, self-esteem, support, or personhood? The question I would like to pose as a further challenge is why we should define change as stressful. What about persons who appraise change as desirable and seek discontinuity? Research that we have conducted with adventure-some elderly who have relocated to the sunbelt (Kahana, Kahana, Segall, Riley, & Vosmik, 1986) consistently underscores the positive response of such individuals to discontinuity and change.

Research on traumatic stress also provides a useful counterpoint to excessive emphasis on appraisals by demonstrating that not all stress is in the eyes of the beholder. Research on extreme stress has demon-strated common and enduring human response to a multiplicity of trauma. In the areas of extreme stress, appraisal plays a lesser role in defining experiences as stressful. The meaning attached to an expe-rience and interpretation of trauma in the context of the total life experience of the older individual, however, may shape the ultimate outcomes of trauma and the ability of the traumatized person for self-healing. Thus, we must remember the overarching impact of stress, while at the same time marvel at individual differences in response.

In addition to the substantive challenges to a totally appraisal-based approach to the stress paradigm, I would like to add a methodological caution arising from focus on measurement. Factor analytical studies in the area of subjective well-being have called attention to the possibility that when we focus on subjective aspects of stress or subjective aspects of support, particularly in the framework of cross-sectional studies, we may be observing spurious associations (Dohrenwend, Dohrenwend, Dodson, & Shrout, 1984). Association between the constructs we measure may not be due to causal linkage or correlation but due to actual overlap in the concepts being measured. Thus, it is possible that the older person exhibiting high morale expresses a generally positive world view by reporting that life events caused only minimal disruption in his or her life and by voicing satisfaction with his or her supports. Thus, the stress "which is in the eyes of the beholder" may be reported through dark-colored or rose-colored glasses.

WHERE DO THE VARIABLES OF SUPPORT, COPING, HEALTH, AND WELL-BEING FIT IN OUR PARADIGM?

In articulating conceptual models of stress and in our empirical studies to test them, there is generally a predictable sequencing of the elements of the model. Stress is typically seen as a stimulus impinging on the older person. Thus, it is the independent variable in our designs.

Psychosocial well-being and health are seen as outcomes or dependent variables in most of stress research. Coping or social supports are generally seen as buffers (mediators or moderators) in this paradigm. One of the exciting contributions of this book has been calling attention to the fruitfulness of alternative sequencing of variables.

Jackson and Antonucci raise this as an intriguing point in this book when they suggest that social support may serve as an insulator against stressful life events. Similarly, it may be useful to move away from a view of coping as a traitlike resource and consider it in a dynamic framework as an evolving skill. Such a view of coping is also compatible with intervention and therapeutic efforts. Our recent research among old-old residents of a Florida retirement community supports the usefulness of reordering the traditional, independent, intervening, and dependent variables in stress research. Although most researchers in the field of aging and stress consider only reactive behaviors of individuals marshalled after the stresses have already arisen, it may be valuable to specify a preventive stress paradigm that considers activities by the elderly that may avert the adverse impact of future stresses.

One promising direction for such inquiry may be the consideration of proactive adaptations among the aged that may prepare them to deal with stresses of late life (Lawton, 1989). Our studies of 1,000 old-old residents of a Florida retirement community suggest that the elderly are prone to engage in both self-enhancing and contributory behaviors that are likely to retard frailty, enhance social resources, and also contribute to subjective well-being (Kahana et al., 1990). Specifically, we noted the high incidence (72%) of regular exercise and other health promotion activities. These elderly also engaged in planning for the future and other self-improvement activities. In addition, helping others, advocacy, and social participation were identified as prevalent proactive behaviors among older respondents. Health promotion is likely to retard the onset of the stress of frailty, whereas other proactive behaviors are likely to generate social supports that may be activated during future times of need.

IS THERE STRESS BEYOND LIFE EVENTS?

Chiriboga aptly notes in this book that stress research has alternatively focused on singular major stressors (which he terms catastrophic stress), life event stress, or everyday hassles. It could thus appear that older persons experience only a given type of stress. Progress in the field of stress research may be defined in terms of specification of the type of stress most important for exploring ill health or psychological distress. Yet, it is evident, based on common sense as well as clinical work with the elderly, that older adults experience the full spectrum of stressors. They endure cumulative life crises throughout their personal history, experience recent life events; encounter chronic stress brought about by ill health, environmental, and social problems; and confront daily hassles.

In considering the impact of stress on the elderly, the independent variables are generally defined as psychosocial stressors or life events that in turn result in physical illness. Yet in the case of the elderly, chronic illness or increased frailty may be considered as major stressors (independent variables) that in turn may result in outcomes of relocation to more sheltered living environments. In fact, disregard of frailty and illness as a major chronic stressor in late life leads us to underestimate old-age specific stressors.

Comprehensive conceptualizations of stress will have to come to terms with the need for measuring and aggregating the full spectrum of stressors that impinge on older adults and that, in combination, contribute to deficits in health and well-being. Accordingly, the observation that stress explains only a relatively small portion of the variance in well-being of the aged may, at least in part, be attributable to the absence of comprehensive and cumulative consideration of stresses experienced. Furthermore, the correct time lag for observing impact of stresses on older adults requires better specification. Even though 1 year is the standard used in life events literature, certain events such as widowhood may express their full impact only after 2 or 3 years. Although studies of late life stress typically consider only one type of stressor, the elderly experience them all. Researchers need to get busy and develop more comprehensive models of stress that allow for enumeration, summation, and, ultimately, integration of the diverse forms and types of stress impinging on the elderly.

WHAT IS THE PROPER UNIT OF ANALYSIS FOR RESEARCH ON STRESS AND AGING?

Although research on stress and aging is generally focused on the older individual, it often does so without actually ascertaining perspectives of the older person. I agree with Hubbard's suggestion that listening to disadvantaged older persons describe the stresses of aging may do a great deal for enhancing our understanding of *stress* and *coping* from the older person's perspective. In fact, we probably need to listen far more to the elderly as informants about their survival skills or crisis management strategies if we are to transcend the sterility of current approaches to the study of stress. If we did so we might not assume that survival skills of the elderly can be ascertained through "Ways of Coping Indexes," which ask elders whether in response to a major stressor they would be very likely, somewhat likely, not very likely, or not at all likely to draw on past experience. In the words of one of our hard-of-hearing institutionalized respondents whom we asked this "profound" question: "I told you already: They *all like me here* and that is all that counts!"

I agree with Chiriboga that our measures of stress must reflect the conceptual understandings we seek. At present, too often, elements of the stress paradigm are defined by existing measures of a variable. Coping scales, as noted earlier, represent a good case in point. Thus, we often conceptualize human adaptation to stress as the separate scores individuals receive on scales that inquire about their likelihood to use a set of coping responses when facing a hypothetical problem situation. Older persons coping with a problem generally use multiple strategies used sequentially or in combination. Accordingly faced with illness of a loved one they may take both problem-focused and emotion-focused actions. They may seek competent medical help in an instrumental fashion, but also feel sad or anxious regarding the possibility of adverse outcomes while waiting for test results. The static and unidimensional measurement strategies currently available thus result in static and unidimensional views of coping. Stress research could benefit greatly if conceptualization were to precede assessment rather than be constrained by existing measures. Furthermore, we may enrich our research by considering coping strategies in a situation-specific and -dynamic fashion rather than only as traitlike or generic responses to all problem situations.

WHY IS STRESS RESEARCH OFTEN CONFUSING?

I almost failed to muster the courage to ask this question, but I was emboldened by incidental comments made by Kasl, and Jackson and

Antonucci in this book about semantic misuses in stress research. Kasl discusses the term *good stress*, which intermittently appears in the literature, and then dismisses it as confusing. Jackson and Antonucci note the term *negative support* and suggest that the term is counterproductive. Stress research and social science research in general have a lot of tolerance for scientific jargon. Yet it is important that we try to keep our terminology simple. If it is good, it is probably not stress. Remarriage in late life viewed in its totality may be good, but it also has stressful components. Marriage, then, is good, but its stressful components are bad.

The case of negative support is similar. For example, Mr. Jones may be getting a lot of help from a doting daughter. It may be too much help, and he may not like feeling dependent. It may be useful to term such support excessive and recognize its negative consequences, but it is not useful to speak of Mr. Jones as getting negative support. Simplifying our terms and ensuring that our efforts to describe complex issues do not result in confusion can go a long way to clear up the paradigm. Semantic confusion based on our need to invent original and evermore complex terms for the phenomena we study thus represents one important and easily remediable source of confusion.

Even as we eschew the temptation to add confusion through jargon, we must recognize that diversity could also masquerade as confusion. If the same pattern of response to stress does not occur in diverse populations, we may have uncovered clarifying clues rather than added confusion. A second step toward reducing confusion may thus come from identifying diversity in responses to stress.

In considering the development of a field, we always have to work hard at the beginning to establish the legitimacy of our orientation and seek coherence and commonalities. In gerontology for many years we focused on what all aged persons have in common. Now that the Gerontological Society has become a large, complex organization; the *Journal of Gerontology* has split in four; and we are official members of an "aging society," the spotlight has increasingly fallen on diversity. I believe that stress research is undergoing a similar evolution. Lieberman's interesting data in this book on the different typologies of adaptation to grief may prove such diversity rather than illustrate the confusing nature of the stress paradigm or pose a serious challenge to its utility.

I do not believe that the concepts considered in the context of the stress paradigm are inherently confusing. It is our failure to define our concepts clearly and our unwillingness to deal forthrightly with the complexities inherent in the phenomena we study that are the likely culprits in the confusion we may encounter. Much of the apparent confusion may thus be eliminated by recognizing complexity and eliminating jargon in an effort to clarify our paradigm.

IS STRESS A STIMULUS OR A RESPONSE, AND IS IT INSIDE OR OUTSIDE THE PERSON?

This book mirrors diversity in orientation to these questions found in the stress literature. Pearlin and Mullan illustrate their position in this book that stress and age are not clearly related by citing data on indicators of stress such as depression and anxiety. In contrast, Boaz Kahana argues that psychological distress does not necessarily accompany experiences of even extreme life stress. These two orientations reflect divergence in definitions of stress as a stimulus or as a response.

The stimulus versus response distinction is useful for understanding divergent findings in stress research and is not necessarily tied to external versus internal views of stress. Accordingly, one might consider physical illness either as a stressor or as a response to stress. In either case, illness is a characteristic or affliction of the individual rather than of his or her environment. Even while we may logically consider external as well as internal stressors impinging on individuals, it is useful to note that the response to stress is definitely an internal rather than external property.

Although the divergence in considerations of stress as internal or external, or stimulus or response may add to the apparent confusion of the paradigm, each approach may be defensible as long as a study is internally consistent. Because authors do not typically explicate the position they take in this regard, it is helpful for consumers of stress research to ask themselves the question: Does the study being considered use internal vs. external, or stimulus vs. response definitions of stress?

WHAT IS THE ROLE OF AGE IN THE STUDY OF STRESS?

Several of the chapters in this book specifically address the issue of relevance of age in the stress paradigm. A major conclusion of Kasl's provocative analysis of methodological parameters of research on stress and aging is the notion that age does not significantly influence the impact of psychosocial factors on health status. This conclusion, by Kasl's own account, appears to be counterintuitive. Yet, to the extent that it is empirically supported, it provides positive challenges to gerontologists to describe and understand the nature and determinants of invulnerability in late life. Future research in the field of stress and aging may provide valuable insights by focusing on late-life vulnerability in the context of the stress paradigm (Kahana, Kahana, & Kinney, 1990). It is possible that reformulation of our traditional approaches in conceptualizing stress and aging may result in new understandings of the ways in which age is salient to stress research. Aldwin's presentation offers such a reformulation pointing to the ways in which the study of stress and aging can serve to enrich our views of human development.

Yet in looking at research published in the gerontological literature and dealing with stresses confronted by older adults, we seldom explicitly ask about the role of age. Gerontological research generally provides an examination of stress, its mediators, and outcomes among various and sundry samples of old people. Age is typically only an implicit variable in gerontological studies. For example, caregiving stress has been studied among spouses of elderly patients, thereby addressing a late-life stressor. Such research may be as much a study of gender as it is of age, with neither variable explicitly modeled. Variability in age is also generally limited among respondents in gerontological studies, which may concern the young-old or old-old without a comparison group of young or middle-aged subjects. When age is included in the analytical scheme of studies of stress health and aging, it is typically treated as a control variable.

Some stress researchers have argued that the elderly are particularly likely to confront losses and other stressful life events at a time when their adaptive capacities have diminished. Others argue that older adults may be more resilient than the young because of accumulated past experiences in dealing with negative events (Norris & Murrell, 1987). To choose systematically between such alternatives, longitudinal studies are needed to address the nature of changes in stress, resources, and health as well as the changing relationships of the components of the stress paradigm at different points in the life cycle.

WHAT DOES IT MEAN IF PEOPLE DO WELL DESPITE STRESSFUL SITUATIONS?

Stress research is attractive because it has action implications and thus relevance to real-life problems of actual people. Yet the stress paradigm allows for alternative assumptions that create some noteworthy ethical dilemmas. If people do well despite problem situations, this could occur because stress is good, or because people are adaptable and can overcome great adversity.

Research in several areas relevant to the elderly has documented remarkable resiliency among older adults. One example of such resiliency relates to work in institutional settings that demonstrated that institutionalized elderly often improve their subjective well-being after institutionalization (Kahana, Kahana, & Young, 1987). Another noteworthy example of resiliency is demonstrated in research on Holocaust survivors who, despite the horrors they endured, appear to show good social adjustment and adaptation to aging. The moral dilemmas posed by such research relate to possible misinterpretation of findings about resiliency as providing justification for placing human beings into stressful or even traumatic situations.

Several of the chapters in this book dealing with intervention point out yet another meaningful response to our question. Kennedy's chapter illustrates the very useful roles that pharmacological and other biomedically oriented treatment approaches can play in assisting individuals to "do well" despite stressful situations that they experience. In fact, the scientific community has just begun to identify some of the important biochemical markers of stress exposure. Explicating the role of biological mechanisms as mediators of the stress process represents a promising and as yet little understood area with great heuristic value for future stress research.

WHY DO BAD THINGS HAPPEN TO GOOD PEOPLE AND IS ANYONE RESPONSIBLE FOR STRESS ENDURED BY ELDERS?

The chapter by Walz and Brown in this book addresses the issue of society's contributions to the stress process and to adaptation of older persons who experienced major stresses. They argue that current public policy that does not facilitate home care of the elderly unnecessarily contributes to the stresses endured by them. Because society's role in the stress process is such an important and neglected aspect of the study of stress, I am taking the liberty of briefly outlining some of the challenges posed by consideration of the ways in which society may shape elements of the stress process. It is my hope that attention directed at society's role may result in addressing these issues more extensively in stress research in the future.

Little is known as yet about the social context of stress and the etiological or protective roles played by society in the development of stressful situations. The role of society in creating stress is particularly salient in man-made disasters and on a lesser scale for role losses encountered by the elderly. There has been little concern in the area of general stress research with social or societal antecedents of stress. Stresses, such as life events, are assumed to be risks of living that are unavoidable. In the area of extreme stress there is greater concern about social or societal factors that form the backdrop to traumatic life situations. Abuse of the elderly may be a case in point, focusing on elderly who are exposed to extreme trauma. Interventions that help remove the causes of such trauma may be just as useful as interventions aimed at mitigating the ill effects of trauma.

It is important to consider the social context of trauma both for reasons of scientific understanding, and also on ethical and moral grounds. Thus, the conceptual framework within which stress research is embedded should not favor paradigms that implicitly or explicitly blame the victims. Gerontological research has increasingly moved from consideration of elders to consideration of caregivers, service providers, and recognition of the importance of social and family context for understanding well-being in late life. Stress research could be greatly enhanced by paying greater attention to the integration of these related elements.

Consideration of the etiologic role of society in stresses experienced by elders represents fertile ground for conceptual development. Although the work of classical sociological theorists from Durkheim to Marx is relevant to broad elements of those etiological roles, we have not succeeded in formulating a taxonomy of the etiological roles of society that is directly relevant to stresses that impinge on older individuals. I have noted earlier in this overview that the stress literature considers stress as a given and does not concern itself with the ways stresses arise. Thus, we may consider a set of life changes or events, such as being a victim of a crime or having problems with one's children, which may cause stress to a person, but we seldom address the question as to whether society or the individual was responsible for these stresses. Societal factors or personal factors that predispose a person or class of persons to victimization or that generate stressful life situations are generally not addressed.

In studying criminal victimization, personal rather than social predisposing factors are generally cited in the victimology literature. Thus, for example, frail elders are said to be more commonly mugged than competent and well elderly. Nevertheless, the etiological relevance of society must also be apparent. Society's role in creating an environment where crimes occur has been noted by feminist scholars regarding victims of rape. Thus, although society is not directly responsible for crimes of the individual rapist, its tolerance of date rapes or wife abuse and its refusal to prosecute perpetrators vigorously may be seen as setting the stage for high rates of violence against women.

The diverse roles played by society at large in relation to stress endured by the elderly range from negative etiological roles to positive preventive roles. They differ in terms of active or passive dimensions and in terms of impact at different stages of the stress process. Specifically, they range from originating roles to contributing roles, revictimizing roles, failure to protect, healing roles, and preventive roles.

Originating roles of society include those situations in which society was the proximate cause of the very occurrence of the traumatic situation and the personal victimization of a given human being. War and instances of genocide are prime examples in this category. Society can also play an indirect *contributing role* to the unfolding of stressful events. The victim or survivor in this case is not directly traumatized by society but by individuals who themselves are victims of social conditions. Accordingly, society may be responsible for poverty, alienation, and dehumanization of citizens, which in turn increase the probability of individual victimization. Another negative role may be played by society in the aftermath of trauma when it *revictimizes* survivors. Social stigma accorded to victims or survivors of stress and trauma exemplifies society's role in maintaining the survivor in a state of continued victimization. Thus, for example, an abused older person may be institutionalized in a misguided effort to protect him or her from the abuser.

Although in the preceding examples societal forces directly or indirectly contributed to the etiology or perpetration of stress, society may also be seen as playing a role in victimization of citizens through failure to protect them from harm. Society's *failure to protect* its citizens from harm is related to its role in the etiology of the trauma. Thus, society has a responsibility to protect citizens from natural disasters as well as acts by its individual members that may cause harm to others. In the case of several recent train wrecks, society may be seen as failing to regulate the workplace in terms of drug testing. Similarly the occurrence of elder abuse in nursing homes may not be directly caused by societal factors. Nevertheless, what Jules Henry (1963) refers to as the "social conscience" is lulled to complacency without exerting meaningful regulatory rules over nursing homes, which would protect frail elders from capricious or uncaring staff and provide them with what may be termed "rightful life."

The role potentially played by society in relation to victims in the aftermath of trauma need not be only a negative one. Avoiding practices or policies that perpetuate stress deals only with the negative half of the spectrum. Society may also play a *healing role* in relation to adverse sequelae of stress. For example, the warm acknowledgment accorded to soldiers returning from the Gulf War may constitue part of such a healing response; in a small and belated way the memorials built to those who perished in Vietnam and the Holocaust similarly promote healing responses. A final important but seldom realized role lies in society's activities toward prevention of stress. Society is generally more prone to take a reactive rather than proactive role in terms of its efforts to protect citizens from stress and trauma.

WHY DO WE KEEP USING THE STRESS PARADIGM IF IT HAS SO MANY PROBLEMS?

Some people might argue that to get funded for our research we must study something that is a problem. The stress paradigm provides a conceptual framework for many problem-centered studies of aging. I do not believe that we use the stress paradigm for such cynical reasons.

On an intellectual level, the stress paradigm remains attractive despite its complexities and ambiguities because it addresses some of the most fundamental questions that have intrigued social and behavioral scientists. The stress model addresses three fundamental questions in social science research: (a) What is the nature of interaction between persons and the environment? (b) What is the linkage between mind and body? (c) To what extent are human beings responders or initiators in their daily behavior? The stress paradigm allows for investigation of interactions between persons and environments by considering conditions that create disequilibrium or incongruence between personal need and environmental press. It allows for determination of physical health consequences of psychological distress and, conversely, it permits examination of the impact of physical illness (a stressor) on subjective well-being. Finally, focus on adverse outcomes subsequent to stress depicts the individual primarily as responder, whereas focus on efforts to cope with stress acknowledges the role of the person as initiator as well as regulator.

On the level of practice and policy one might ask if there is anything in the stress paradigm itself or the related research that arises from it that informs us about helping the elderly. Part of the answer to this question is that in stress research, just as in most other social research, researchers seldom concern themselves with translating their findings into systematic guidelines for practice. Furthermore, there is a tendency for practice and policy to develop independently of research influenced by availability of funding or other political considerations. Nevertheless, Gatz's chapter in this book provides an excellent example of careful conceptualization serving to define useful strategies of intervention. Not only are existing conceptual frameworks applied selectively to practice issues, but a comprehensive approach to intervention must grow out of a comprehensive conceptual model. Gatz's demonstration of the relevance of each element of the stress paradigm for practice and intervention underscores the appeal and utility of the stress model.

On a moral or ethical level, the stress paradigm permits us to consider intervention to protect elders from stress or to help them cope with unavoidable stress or its consequences. Thus, it allows us to integrate our motivation as do-gooders who are interested in enhancing quality of life for the elderly with our stance as scientists interested in better understanding and exploring social phenomena.

IS IT WHOM WE KNOW OR IS IT WHAT WE KNOW THAT SHAPES OUR UNDERSTANDING OF STRESS RESEARCH?

To what extent are understandings, presented in this book or elsewhere in stress research, shaped by selection of investigators and their specialized orientations? Putting on my hat as one of the editors of this book, I can say with conviction that we strived for balance and diversity in chapters. At the same time, editing a book is never a totally impersonal or objective process. Editors' awareness of research in the field is limited at the very least by the scope of their socialization, readings, disciplinary boundaries, and reliance on national and international perspectives.

Furthermore, the understandings gained in the field of stress research are also shaped by orientations of researchers. Thus, for example, Pearlin and Mullan aptly point out in this book that specialization of research by age groups studied has influenced what we know about the relationship of age and stress. There are separate bodies of research that consider stress in children, adolescents, young adults, and among older adults. Researchers focusing on each of these groups tend to emphasize those life experiences that have been found problematic by the particular age group they study.

A further selection bias shaping our understandings relates to the tendency of each contributor to a book such as this one to highlight his or her own research in the context of a synthesis of the field. Although on the one hand this can be illuminating, it can also be misleading. In a journal article that reports on a particular study, it is clear to the reader that the author reports on a singular work. In contrast, in a critical review of a literature we expect an unbiased synthesis of insights gained across diverse investigations. In compendiums, such as the present one, experts in the field tend to review their own program of research. Typically, they do so without specifying parameters or limitations within which their own research program operates.

Reader beware! What we know is definitely shaped by whom we know.

DOES THE DEVELOPMENTAL STAGE OF THE FIELD SHAPE OUR RESEARCH ON STRESS AND AGING?

I would like to conclude this overview by considering the potential role of the age and stage of our research efforts in shaping our approaches to stress research. This discussion is related to the issue of stages in the study of stress addressed by Chiriboga. He classifies early work as reflecting a catastrophe model, whereas later stages reflect on life events and finally focus on stresses of everyday life. The challenge to stress research in Chiriboga's view is integration of these three different approaches. Piaget's characterization of individual human development as progressing in the direction of increasing differentiation and hierarchical integration also provides a useful model for considering the evolution of research in the field of stress and aging.

School-age children approach problem solving in ways that characterized early work in stress research and aging. During the early phase of our studies, we dutifully did our homework and conducted careful, diligent but uncritical studies that followed examples provided by researchers in the field of general stress research. Thus, we slowly chipped away at questions posed by general stress research. We next moved to an adolescent stage of rebellion and proceeded to question the utility of the entire stress paradigm as we discovered that the models presented to us by the field were not always workable or applicable. As we approached middle adulthood, we reflected on the limitations of alternative stress models and recognized that the stress paradigm is not entirely useless after all.

Research focusing on adaptation of the aged has underscored the interconnectedness of problems faced by older adults that on the surface appeared unique and not readily subsumed in a stress framework. We now appreciate the complexities inherent in problems, variables, and measurement approaches and are slowly rediscovering valuable roots in early work relevant to the study of health, stress, and late-life adaptation. As our field matures further and we enter late life, we may need to conserve our energy a bit; it is hoped that this will cause us to seek greater parsimony in our explanations. As part of our life review, we may be able to integrate insights gained from earlier studies with our current discoveries, and we may look hopefully toward achievements yet to come from a new generation of research or even from a new generation of researchers.

We may thus come to realize that one of the greatest dangers to any field of scientific study is routinization of inquiry or blinders to fresh insights. I have come away from editing this book with many fresh insights about the role of stress in late life and the broader stress paradigm. I hope that readers of this volume will also have found new questions as well as new answers in the work that has been shared by contributors to this book.

REFERENCES

Dohrenwend, B. S., Dohrenwend, B. P., Dodson, M., & Shrout, P. (1984). Symptoms, hassles, social supports, and life events: Problem of confounded measures. *Journal of Abnormal Psychology, 93*, 222–230.

Folkman, S., & Lazarus, R. S. (1980). An analysis of coping in a middle-aged community sample. *Journal of Health and Social Behavior, 21*, 219–239.

Henry, J. (1963). *Culture against man.* New York: Random House.

Kahana, B., Kahana, E., & Kinney, J. M. (1990). Coping among vulnerable elders. In Z. Harel, P. Ehrlich, & R. Hubbard (Eds.), *The vulnerable aged: People, services, and policies* (pp. 64–85). New York: Springer.

Kahana, E., Kahana, B., Segall, M., Riley, K., & Vosmik, J. (1986). Motivators, resources and barriers in voluntary international migration of the elderly: The Case of Israel-bound aged. *Cross-Cultural Gerontology, 1*, 191–208.

Kahana, E., Kahana, B., & Young, R. (1987). Influences of diverse stresses on health and well-being of community aged. In A. M. Fowler (Ed.), *Post-traumatic stress: The healing journey.* Washington, DC: Veterans' Administration.

Kahana, E., Kahana, B., Stange, K., Novatney, J., Borawski, E., & Kercher, K. (1990, November). *Proactive lifestyles and invulnerability to stresses of frailty among the old-old living in retirement communities.* Presented at the annual meeting of the Gerontological Society of America, Boston.

Lawton, M. P. (1989). Environmental proactivity and affect in older people. In S. Spacapan & S. Oskamp (Eds.), *The Social Psychology of Aging* (pp. 135–163). Newbury Park, CA: Sage.

Norris, F. N., & Murrell, S. A. (1987). Older adult family stress and adaptation before and after bereavement. *Journal of Gerontology, 42*, 606–612.

Wethington, E., & Kessler, R. C. (1986). Perceived support, received support, and adjustment to stressful life events. *Journal of Health and Social Behavior, 27*, 78–89.

Index